# GYNAECOLOGICAL SYMPTOMS
## IN PRIMARY CARE

# Gynaecological Symptoms in Primary Care

ROBERT HAMMOND
FRCS, MRCOG
Consultant Obstetrician and Gynaecologist
University Hospital, Nottingham

AND

MICHAEL McGHEE
DRCOG, MRCGP, MFFP
GP trainer,
Nottingham Vocational Training Scheme
Instructing Doctor in Family Planning
and Foundation Member
of the Faculty of Family Planning
and Reproductive Health Care
of the Royal College of Obstetricians
and Gynaecologists

Blackwell
Science

© 1996 by
Blackwell Science Ltd
Editorial Offices:
Osney Mead, Oxford OX2 0EL
25 John Street, London WC1N 2BL
23 Ainslie Place, Edinburgh EH3 6AJ
238 Main Street, Cambridge
  Massachusetts 02142, USA
54 University Street, Carlton
  Victoria 3053, Australia

Other Editorial Offices:
  224, Boulevard Saint Germain
  75007 Paris, France

Blackwell Wissenschafts-Verlag GmbH
  Kurfürstendamm 57
  10707 Berlin, Germany

Zehetnergasse 6
A-1140 Wien, Austria

First published 1996

Set by Excel Typesetters, Hong Kong
Printed and bound in Great Britain
at the Alden Press Ltd, Oxford and
Northampton

The Blackwell Science logo is a
trade mark of Blackwell Science Ltd,
registered at the United Kingdom
Trade Marks Registry

A catalogue record for this title
is available from the British Library

ISBN 0-86542-679-1

DISTRIBUTORS

Marston Book Services Ltd
PO Box 269
Abingdon, Oxon OX14 4YN
(Orders: Tel: 01235 465500
          Fax: 01235 465555)

USA
Blackwell Science, Inc.
238 Main Street
Cambridge, MA 02142
(Orders: Tel: 800 215-1000
          617 876-7000
          Fax: 617 492-5263)

Canada
Copp Clark, Ltd
2775 Matheson Blvd East
Mississauga, Ontario
Canada, L4W 4P7
(Orders: Tel: 800 263-4374
          905 238-6074)

Australia
Blackwell Science Pty Ltd
54 University Street
Carlton, Victoria 3053
(Orders: Tel: 03 9347-0300
          Fax: 03 9349-3016)

Library of Congress
Cataloging-in-Publication Data

Hammond, Robert, MRCOG.
  Gynaecological symptoms in
  primary care/Robert Hammond
  and Michael McGhee.
       p.      cm.
  Includes bibliographical references
  and index.
  ISBN 0-86542-679-1
  1. Generative organs, Female—
Diseases. 2. Physicians (General
practice) I. McGhee, M. F. II. Title.
  [DNLM: 1. Genital Diseases,
  Female—diagnosis. 2. Primary
  Health Care.
  WP141 H227g 1996]
RG101.H28 1996
618.1—dc20
DNLM/DLC                    95-51671
for Library of Congress         CIP

# Contents

# Preface

Gynaecological symptoms account for up to 20% of all consultations in general practice. Menstrual irregularities, pelvic pain, dysuria and frequency of micturition are all regularly encountered. About one in six couples seek specialist help because of difficulty in conceiving and much useful preliminary investigation can be done by the general practitioner before referral. Vaginal discharge affects women of all ages and accounts for 7% of all consultations in general practice yet there is still wide variation in its management. More miscarriages take place at home than are admitted to hospital. These and many other areas of gynaecological practice have considerable areas of overlap between hospital gynaecology units and primary care.

Training in gynaecology is, however, hospital based, with inadequate undergraduate teaching, which rarely reflects presenting symptomatology, concentrating more on theory than practice. Traditional gynaecology textbooks are disease orientated with little attention to presenting symptoms, and not always easy to interpret in the clinical setting in which they present.

This book aims to cover most areas of gynaecology as they present in primary care. It is written by a consultant gynaecologist in a teaching hospital and an experienced principal in general practice, who is also a vocational trainer. The topics chosen and the style of presentation are intended to make reference easy and practical. The book should appeal not only to principals and registrars in general practice but also to final year medical students and new senior house officers.

This book uses the knowledge and experience of its two authors to bring together the sort of practical information which will make the management of gynaecological symptoms within general practice more methodical and complete, to the benefit of the patient and doctor alike.

R. Hammond

M.F. McGhee

# 1: Menstrual Disorders

Abnormal premenopausal vaginal bleeding is the commonest reason for referral to a gynaecology out-patient clinic. It is a major cause of morbidity and accounts for a considerable amount of time lost from work. In a large number of cases the aetiology is hormonal imbalance and is thus labelled 'dysfunctional bleeding', which is defined as abnormal uterine bleeding in the absence of any pathological cause. It is by definition a diagnosis of exclusion. Pregnancy must be the first consideration as a cause of abnormal vaginal bleeding in a woman still in her reproductive years. Beta-human chorionic gonadotrophin (HCG) assays are now so sensitive that a negative (serum) test excludes pregnancy.

## Symptoms

The exact pattern of the abnormal bleeding, including timing within the cycle, date of onset and periodicity should be carefully recorded as well as whether the periods are regular or heavy. Regular heavy periods are virtually never due to potentially life-threatening conditions unless they are associated with intermenstrual bleeding (IMB). Postcoital bleeding (PCB) is an important symptom and may be caused by serious cervical pathology especially cervical carcinoma. Reported heavy blood loss is subjective but the passing of large clots is supportive evidence. Completely irregular bleeding may be indicative of serious pathology including malignancy anywhere in the genital tract but most especially the cervix, endometrium or ovary.

Other associated symptoms may be suggestive of certain conditions. Pain is often associated with menorrhagia due to fibroids or endometriosis. In endometriosis the pain often begins prior to the period and eases with the onset of bleeding.

1

Pain in combination with irregular bleeding or discharge may be caused by pelvic infection.

Current and past contraceptive practice should be enquired into. All types of hormonal contraception may cause irregular bleeding and the presence of an intrauterine contraceptive device (IUCD) may be associated with both irregular bleeding and menorrhagia. Symptoms of both pregnancy and the menopause should be sought wherever appropriate.

Abnormal bleeding may arise from conditions outside the pelvis. Endocrine disorders in the hypothalamus, pituitary, thyroid and adrenal glands may all cause menstrual problems as well as generalized bleeding disorders. A careful history therefore of any unusual bleeding or bruising, or delay in stopping bleeding after a cut or tooth extraction are all relevant. Finally, recent weight change, particularly in association with galactorrhoea or hirsutism should be noted.

## Signs

A careful general examination, looking in particular for extrapelvic disease, should be performed paying particular attention to the breasts and thyroid gland. Clinical assessment of anaemia can be misleading and in cases of any doubt a full blood count should be taken. Abdominal examination may reveal tenderness in association with infection or endometriosis and a mass arising out of the pelvis will most commonly be due to a large fibroid or ovarian pathology.

Vaginal examination with a speculum will disclose cervical lesions such as carcinoma, a polyp or ectropion. Likewise the threads of an IUCD should be visible if there is a coil *in situ* and if they are not, gentle probing of the cervix with an Emmat thread retriever should be carefully attempted. If this is not successful an ultrasound scan of the pelvis should be arranged. An offensive vaginal discharge is suggestive of pelvic infection and high vaginal and endocervical swabs should be taken for culture and separate specimens should be taken for chlamydial culture. Endometriomas are occasionally seen on the cervix or in the vaginal fornices.

Following speculum examination, a bimanual vaginal examination should be performed. The cervix should be felt and its regularity and consistency assessed. Cervical excitation (tenderness on lateral movement of the cervix) is suggestive of pelvic infection. The size of the uterus, its position and mobility should all be noted as well as any tenderness, as should any tenderness or masses in the fornices.

## Investigations

A full blood count, thyroid function tests and serum follicle-stimulating hormone (FSH), luteinizing hormone (LH) and beta-HCG may be appropriate, as may swabs and a cervical smear as indicated above. A normal cervical smear does not exclude a cervical abnormality because there is a significant false negative rate.

Ultrasound examination of the pelvis is useful in assessing uterine size as well as the presence of extrauterine lesions such as tubal collections, ovarian masses and free fluid within the pelvis.

## Management

Management will be determined by the evaluation of the history, examination and special investigations where appropriate. In the majority of cases the provisional diagnosis will be dysfunctional uterine bleeding (DUB) and the management will then be determined by the type of bleeding and the age of the patient.

### Regular heavy periods

In cases of regular heavy periods, at any age, the treatment options are as follows.

**1** Non-hormonal medical treatment, e.g. prostaglandin antagonist or antifibrinolytic agents, e.g. Dicynene.
**2** Hormonal medical treatment, e.g. progestogens, the oral contraceptive pill or hormone replacement therapy.
**3** Surgical treatment. Endometrial resection or laser ablation of the endometrium, or hysterectomy.

Hysteroscopic examination of the endometrial cavity with biopsy or dilatation and curettage (D&C) has no place in the management of this group except in the assessment of suitability for endoscopic destruction of the endometrium. The risk of endometrial malignancy in this group of patients is very low. Medical treatment has a good chance of success and non-hormonal therapy carries less side-effects than hormonal treatment.

The surgical options are not compatible with retention of fertility. Sterilization may be appropriate at the same time as endometrial resection. The advantages of endometrial resection over hysterectomy are a shorter length of time in hospital, quicker recovery and no abdominal scar. The disadvantages are that it rarely results in complete amenorrhoea, the long-term effect has yet to be assessed and the likelihood of success in patients experiencing pain with periods is small.

*Irregular periods ± IMB ± PCB*

In cases of irregular periods ± IMB ± PCB in women aged less than 40 years the treatment options are as follows.
**1** Initial trial of hormonal therapy for three months. If this is successful discontinue the treatment and observe. If the problem recurs undertake hysteroscopy and D&C to exclude significant pathology.
**2** If after hysteroscopy and D&C the problem persists, further hormonal treatment may be appropriate *or* endoscopic destruction of the endometrium may be undertaken *or* hysterectomy.

The incidence of endometrial cancer under the age of 40 years is very low, hence hormonal intervention in a pragmatic way to begin with is reasonable, resorting to D&C only if the problem persists. Dilatation and curettage has never been shown to have any therapeutic effect except in stopping an episode of prolonged heavy bleeding which may be necessary in a woman with dysfunctional bleeding. Up to 30% of the endometrium may be left undisturbed during D&C which is becoming superseded by hysteroscopic examination of the endometrium with directed biopsy.

*In cases of irregular periods ± IMB ± PCB in women over the age of 40 years, hysteroscopy and biopsy or D&C are mandatory as the incidence of endometrial carcinoma rises dramatically in this age group.*

## Fibroids

Fibroids are generally associated with painful and heavy periods. If the periods are irregular or associated with intermenstrual bleeding, there may be an additional problem and endometrial biopsy should be considered especially in women over the age of 40 years.

If the uterus is not significantly enlarged by the fibroids, a trial of non-hormonal medical therapy may be worthwhile, e.g. Dicynene. If, however, the uterus is more than the size of an eight-week pregnancy, medical treatment is unlikely to be successful and surgical treatment should be offered. Endoscopic destruction is unlikely to confer any benefit unless the fibroids are small. The type of surgery offered will also be influenced by the woman's wish to retain fertility. Myomectomy may be associated with heavy bleeding and occasionally hysterectomy has to be undertaken to control the bleeding. In addition the uterus may be distorted following the procedure and infection and adhesions are an occasional complication. Fibroids may not only impair fertility but may also be associated with miscarriage and problems later in pregnancy. Prior to performing a myomectomy and occasionally prior to hysterectomy, luteinizing hormone-releasing hormone (LH-RH) analogues may be used to shrink fibroids and hence reduce intra-operative blood loss. The use of these agents, however, has no place in the longer term management of fibroids and the definitive treatment remains hysterectomy.

## Endometriosis and pelvic inflammatory disease

These diagnoses may be suggested by the presence of pelvic tenderness associated with uterine fixation with or without adnexal masses. Appropriate swabs should be taken at the time of examination and laparoscopy may be used to confirm the diagnosis.

Recurrent pelvic infections may be treated with intermittent courses of antibiotics. However, chronic infection often results in continuous pelvic pain increasingly unresponsive to antibiotics and analgesics. The only effective treatment in such cases is surgical clearance of the pelvis including the ovaries. This may be a difficult decision to make as the women are often young and may not yet have had children; however, they are almost always infertile.

The management of endometriosis depends upon the extent of the disease and the individual's wish to reproduce. In severe cases the only effective treatment is pelvic clearance with removal of the ovaries. However, less invasive surgery may be possible and appropriate such as ovarian cystectomy, freeing of adhesions or destruction of endometriotic deposits with diathermy or laser. Less severe cases are usually managed medically by suppressing ovarian function for a few months. The disease may then become quiescent or disappear completely. First line treatment is with high dose progestogens or the oral contraceptive pill; if this is unsuccessful, Danazol or LH-RH analogues may be used, although these are more expensive and have more side-effects.

**Table 1.1** Indications for gynaecological referral due to menstrual disorders.

| | |
|---|---|
| Regular heavy periods, any age | Refer if medical treatment fails |
| Irregular periods ± IMB, ±PCB age less than 40 years | Refer if medical treatment fails after three months |
| Irregular periods ± IMB, ±PCB age greater than 40 years | Refer immediately due to risk of endometrial malignancy |

± IMB, intermenstrual bleeding; ± PCB, postcoital bleeding.

Pregnancy is an excellent treatment for endometriosis.

## Contraceptive problems

If the menstrual disturbance is thought to be related to the coil or oral contraceptive pill then a change of contraception to a barrier method for a few months may be appropriate. Alternatively, if the problem is break-through bleeding, whilst taking a low-dose pill, then a change to a higher dose pill for a few months may rectify matters.

## Cervical lesions

A polyp or ectropion causing postcoital or intermenstrual bleeding may be treated initially to see if the problem resolves. If it does not resolve then the management should follow those of dysfunctional bleeding (see above) with recourse to endometrial biopsy if appropriate and certainly in all cases where the patient is aged over 40 years. An ectropion should only be destroyed if the patient has had a recent negative cervical smear as diathermy or laser treatment of an ectropion may compromise future cervical assessment.

The presence of an obvious or suspected cervical malignancy should be pursued as a matter of urgency with appropriate examination and biopsy (see Chapter 9).

*Ovarian lesions*

A small ovarian cyst (less than 5 cm in diameter) may be managed by laparoscopy initially and, if thought to be simple, may be aspirated and the contents examined cytologically. If the cyst recurs it should be removed, this may be possible by laparoscopy or an open procedure may be necessary.

Any cyst larger than 5 cm should be removed. If the cyst appears malignant the correct management is pelvic clearance with appropriate additional surgery (see Chapter 9). There is a high incidence of abnormal uterine bleeding in oestrogen secreting tumours, and even in epithelial tumours, almost one-fifth of patients present with abnormal bleeding.

## Questions

**Q1**: When are gonadotrophin-releasing factor (GnRH) analogues indicated?

**A**: GnRH analogues are extremely effective at switching off the ovaries, and therefore switching off menstruation totally. They are useful when all other measures have failed and a woman is continuing to bleed very heavily.

They are also useful, again as a last resort in the management of premenstrual syndrome (PMS), when they can be extremely effective especially in combination with an oestrogen patch to give a steady oestrogen level.

**Q2**: When is laser ablation of the endometrium indicated?

**A**: Laser ablation is indicated for the treatment of menorrhagia but may be less helpful in the management of dysmenorrhoea.

**Q3**: When is hysterectomy by laparoscopy indicated and appropriate?

**A**: Hysterectomy by laparoscopy is attractive in offering a speedy operation and release from hospital by the patient in two to three days only. Unfortunately complications including accidental bladder and ureteric damage, mean that it is still under scrutiny as an alternative to abdominal hysterectomy. If vaginal hysterectomy is possible, this would be the preferred method.

# 2: Urinary Problems

Urinary problems, in particular urinary incontinence, cause considerable suffering in the female population. Many patients do not present to the doctor, perhaps because of the belief that little can be done to improve or help the problem. There are several different types of incontinence and a correct diagnosis is necessary before embarking upon appropriate treatment. Incontinence may be classified as follows.

1 Genuine stress incontinence.
2 Detrusor instability.
3 Overflow incontinence.
4 Fistulae.
5 Neurological causes.
6 Psychogenic causes.
7 Congenital causes.

The first two, genuine stress incontinence and detrusor instability, are by far the most common types of incontinence in gynaecological practice, with overflow and fistulae presenting less frequently. Neurological causes such as multiple sclerosis are rare but should be considered in atypical cases. Congenital problems such as ectopic ureteric implantations usually present to paediatricians. Psychogenic causes can only be diagnosed by exclusion.

## Genuine stress incontinence

### Symptoms

Genuine stress incontinence is due to a weakness of the voluntary sphincter at the level of the internal urethral meatus and may be associated with vaginal prolapse, although not always. It occurs when the intravesical pressure exceeds the urethral pressure and results in involuntary loss of urine. The patient describes sudden leakage of urine on coughing, sneezing, running, jumping or other forms of physical exertion, even during intercourse. This is the only symptom of genuine stress incontinence and in the absence of any other urinary symptoms this is the most likely diagnosis in 95% of patients. However, similar symptoms may be described in association with detrusor instability or overflow incontinence.

*Signs*

Abdominal palpation may reveal an over-distended bladder which may suggest overflow. The patient should be asked to void and then a catheter passed to check the 'residual volume'. Overflow incontinence is an absolute contraindication to surgery for genuine stress incontinence. The patient should then be examined in the standing, lying and left lateral positions. She should be asked to cough and leakage of urine observed. Descent of anterior or posterior vaginal walls should be observed and finally a pelvic examination should be performed to exclude a pelvic mass.

*Investigations*

If symptoms are those as described, and the residual volume is normal, further investigation is not essential. The diagnosis may be confirmed however by visualizing the bladder neck using video-cystourethrography, at a time of increased intravesical pressure. Detrusor instability, which may be associated with genuine stress incontinence, is best demonstrated with subtracted cystometry (see below).

*Management*

In mild genuine stress incontinence, pelvic floor exercises plus treatment such as interferential therapy, a form of ultrasound, may improve the tone of the pelvic floor muscles and improve symptoms.

In more significant cases surgery may be appropriate. Traditional vaginal operations, involving anterior colporrhaphy combined with buttressing of the bladder neck to achieve elevation of the bladder neck at the level of the internal sphincter, are being superseded by abdominal or combined abdominal and vaginal operations. The Burch colposuspension uses an abdominal approach, elevating the bladder neck by suturing the vaginal skin to the ileopectineal ligaments on both sides. This does require some give in the anterior vaginal wall and it may be more appropriate in an elderly woman with an atrophic vagina to perform a Stamey colposuspension using a combined abdominal and vaginal approach to elevate the bladder neck.

Because the bladder neck is raised during all of these procedures, there is increased resistance to voiding afterwards and the bladder must be drained suprapubically until residual volumes are consistently below 100 ml.

Surgery is less likely to succeed in obese patients. Weight loss itself, where appropriate, may relieve the symptoms of genuine stress incontinence.

### Detrusor instability

#### Symptoms

Detrusor instability may result in a number of different symptoms with incontinence often described as a sudden urge to pass urine and an inability to make it to the toilet on time. The urgency is usually combined with frequency which may be related to decreasing bladder size and increasing fear of having an accident. One of the most suggestive symptoms of an unstable bladder is frequent nocturia, which is much less common in psychogenic causes.

Detrusor instability is due to inappropriate contraction of the detrusor muscles in response to increasingly small volumes of urine in the bladder. A vicious circle then ensues with the patient becoming increasingly unable to hold smaller and smaller quantities of urine and experiencing increased frequency and urgency as a result. The bladder ultimately becomes increasingly contracted with marked thickening of the bladder wall. Fortunately most patients do not reach this late stage.

### Signs

Examination often reveals no positive findings although one may demonstrate stress incontinence after coughing; this may result in detrusor stimulation followed by a loss of urine which is said to be slightly delayed in comparison with genuine stress incontinence.

### Investigations

Frequency and urgency even in the absence of dysuria, merits a mid-stream sample of urine for culture and sensitivity.

Bladder pressure studies are required to demonstrate increasing detrusor pressure during bladder filling. Subtracted cystometry involves filling the bladder with saline through a giving set and catheter whilst pressure transducers situated within the bladder record the changing pressures. A rectal pressure transducer records the intra-abdominal pressure which is subtracted from the intravesical pressure to give the true detrusor pressure during filling. In the normal bladder the detrusor pressure should remain low and not start to rise until a large volume of fluid is present, often greater than 500 ml. In an unstable bladder the detrusor pressure may rise gradually with small volumes or may have spikes of pressure increase during filling. The volume at which the first desire to void occurs should be noted as should any leakage, and the final capacity should be recorded. It is often reduced.

## Management

Bladder training and the use of drugs to inhibit detrusor activity are the mainstays of treatment of an unstable bladder. Bladder training involves strict recording of times of voiding, with volumes, and is structured in such a way that the bladder is emptied at a set time interval regardless of the desire to void, gradually increasing the interval until it is acceptable. The drugs most commonly used are the anticholinergic agents which block the passage of impulses at the neuromuscular junction. The dose is titrated against its effect and side-effects, the most common being dry mouth and occasional dizziness on standing. Glaucoma may be precipitated. Calcium channel blockers may also be used for their direct effect on muscle contraction.

In cases where the bladder capacity is low after subtracted cystometry, it is often helpful to perform cystoscopy to assess bladder capacity under anaesthesia in an attempt to improve the bladder response to training and drugs by stretching the bladder. In-patient bladder training is often successful in reducing frequency of micturition but the increased frequency often recurs on discharge.

Where patients have had long-standing detrusor instability and thickening of the bladder wall is demonstrated at cystoscopy, surgery may be necessary such as 'Clam cystoplasty' which incorporates caecum into the bladder or ultimately a urinary diversion with wet or dry stomata.

In patients with a mixture of detrusor instability and genuine stress incontinence, long-term results are usually better if the former is dealt with prior to treatment of the latter.

## Overflow incontinence

### *Symptoms*

Although relatively uncommon in the female, compared with prostatic hypertrophy in the male, failure to make the diagnosis of overflow incontinence may have devastating consequences with back pressure on the kidneys leading to renal failure and ultimately death.

Symptoms are often similar to those of genuine stress incontinence with leakage of urine on exertion. There may be constant dribbling of urine as the large volumes contained in a chronically distended bladder gradually increase. Frequency and urgency are rarely a problem as bladder sensitivity is considerably reduced. Hesitancy, with a feeling of incomplete bladder emptying, and a need to go to the toilet again immediately after micturition, may be present. There may also be leakage of urine on standing following apparent emptying of the bladder.

### *Signs*

Examination of the abdomen may reveal a smoothly enlarged mass arising from the pelvis which is not tender. Vaginal examination may demonstrate apparent stress incontinence.

There may be resistance to passing a catheter if the cause of the problem is a urethral stricture.

### *Investigations*

The diagnosis of overflow incontinence is made by measuring the residual volume after micturition which may be very high. Another useful measurement is urine flow rate.

A mid-stream sample of urine is mandatory as there has been urinary stasis.

Renal ultrasound should be performed as well as biochemical assessment of urinary function.

## Management

Cystoscopy should be performed to inspect and drain the bladder and assess the calibre of the urethra. If the urethra is narrowed then dilatation should be performed at the same time. The bladder should then be kept empty for several days by means of a suprapubic catheter in an attempt to regain muscle tone within the bladder. Any infection present should be treated appropriately. After about a week of free drainage the catheter is clamped and a smooth muscle stimulant such as carbachol is administered to try and achieve satisfactory bladder emptying. If residual volumes remain high the catheter may be left on free drainage for a longer period of time but if still unsuccessful intermittent self-catheterization or a long-term indwelling catheter are the only options.

## Urinary fistulae

### Symptoms

The majority of urinary fistulae are the result of previous surgery. A few are seen in malignant disease and following childbirth.

The cardinal symptom is continuous uncontrolled urinary incontinence. The patient may or may not go to the toilet normally depending upon the size and position of the fistula.

### Signs

The presence of a pool of urine at the vaginal vault is highly suggestive of a fistula and it may be possible to visualize the site.

### Investigations

In cases of doubt the three swab test may be employed. Three cotton wool balls are placed in the vagina one above the other whilst blue dye is injected into the bladder via a urethral catheter. The swabs are removed and their staining with dye will confirm the presence of a fistula and may suggest its position. Cystoscopy should also be performed with radiological investigation of both the bladder and ureters.

## Management

This will depend upon the aetiology and site of the fistula. Surgery should be undertaken by an experienced surgeon as the first attempt is the most likely to be successful. In fistulae due to malignancy, repair is often not possible and symptomatic treatment or urinary diversion are the treatments of choice.

## Haematuria

The presence of frank haematuria or persistent microscopic haematuria in the absence of infection should be investigated by cystoscopy and intravenous pyelography (IVP), particularly to exclude malignancy.

## Dysuria and infections

Urinary tract infections are more common in women than in men due to the shorter urethra and its proximity to the vagina and perineum. Appropriate antibiotic therapy should be commenced.

Some women develop persistent or recurrent infections and should be investigated with cystoscopy and IVP. Sometimes long-term antibiotics are necessary even where no obvious source of infection is found.

Some patients who experience recurrent cystitis without detectable infection may benefit from cystoscopy as well as taking alkylating agents and liberal fluids.

# 3: Infertility

Infertility is a major cause of gynaecological referral and has become established as a sub-specialty amongst gynaecologists. It is responsible for considerable morbidity and affects up to 15% of couples during their reproductive years. There are numerous causes of infertility and a sensible and logical approach to the problem is necessary to minimize the emotional trauma which the couple are subjected to.

The investigation and management of fertility problems is time-consuming and it is important to state this fact to the couple at the first consultation. A general gynaecological clinic may not be the most appropriate setting for consultations and a separate infertility clinic, if available, is ideal. It is also helpful if the same doctor is involved throughout the course of investigations. Physicians dealing with fertility problems should be honest with their patients and not give false or unrealistic hope, or pursue fruitless investigations when it may be more appropriate to advise other options such as adoption.

One-third of cases of subfertility are due to female factors, one-third due to male factors and the remaining one-third due to a combination of male and female problems. It is therefore necessary to investigate both partners before instigating any treatment. In some cases simple advice regarding frequency and timing of intercourse may be all that is required to achieve a successful pregnancy; indeed occasionally psychosexual counselling may sometimes by more appropriate than extensive investigation.

Much of the initial management of subfertile couples can be carried out in the primary healthcare setting, and a good relationship with the general practitioner is highly desirable and possibly even of therapeutic value. The major causes of subfertility are male factors, female factors relating to ovulation and factors involving transport problems.

## Male factors

Male infertility may be due to pre-testicular, testicular or post-testicular causes, but one-third of cases are idiopathic.

### History

The most important question to ask is whether the male partner has been responsible for any pregnancies either with his current or previous partners. Other relevant information should include factors which may adversely affect semen, namely:

1 occupation;
2 age;
3 drug history including Salazopyrin, alcohol and drug abuse;
4 previous infections such as mumps, urinary tract infection or sexually transmitted diseases (STDs);
5 previous surgery such as testicular torsion, orchidopexy, varicocele repair or vasectomy;
6 frequency of intercourse and any problems.

### Examination

Although this is rarely abnormal it is nevertheless important. The general health as well as examination of the external genitalia, lower abdomen and groin is essential.

### Investigation

Urinalysis is cheap and easy to exclude diabetes.

Examination of a freshly produced semen sample after three days without ejaculation. An abnormal result should be followed up with a repeat analysis. Poor motility is an indication to check for anti-sperm antibodies in the serum, particularly following a reversal of vasectomy.

Low sperm counts are an indication for further specialized tests including motility, penetration and fusion. Azoospermia may be due to non-production of sperms or due to a blockage between the testis and external urethral meatus. Follicle-stimulating hormone (FSH) and luteinizing hormone (LH) should be measured and if they are high then there is no action to be taken. If, however, they are normal then a testicular biopsy will be required to establish the presence of sperms. Radiological examination of the vas deferens may be performed to establish whether surgical by-pass is appropriate.

Following vasectomy, microsurgical epididymal sperm aspiration with *in vitro* fertilization is occasionally attempted when re-anastomosis has failed, although the sperm quality may be impaired. In addition anti-sperm antibodies may have developed.

## Female factors

### Ovulation

*History*

Enquire into previous pregnancies with the same or another partner. Enquire into menstrual pattern, if the cycles are regular ovulation is probably taking place. Irregular cycles probably indicate anovulation. Anovulation may occur in polycystic ovarian syndrome (POS), prolactin secreting pituitary adenomas, and in disorders of thyroid function. Enquire into recent weight changes. Enquire into any increase in body hair, particularly of a male distribution (POS) or discharge from nipples (hyperprolactinaemia). Less common causes of anovulation include diabetes and chronic renal failure.

A history of usage of hormonal contraception may be relevant and post-pill amenorrhoea is common. Anovulation following cessation of the oral contraceptive pill usually corrects itself spontaneously within one year.

## Examination

This is often unremarkable. However a bradycardia and enlarged thyroid gland may suggest hypothyroidism whilst breast examination may reveal galactorrhoea. Attention should be made to hair distribution and weight, especially any recent significant change in weight, either loss or gain. Pelvic examination is usually normal but sometimes vaginismus is noted suggesting psychosexual counselling may be appropriate.

## Investigation

FSH, LH, prolactin and thyroid function tests, together with plasma progesterone in the mid-secretory phase to confirm ovulation. Transvaginal ultrasound will identify ovarian follicles and polycystic ovaries.

Recording basal body temperature is notoriously unreliable and may do more harm than good.

## Transport problems

### History

Although most transport problems will be due to tubal factors it is important to establish that satisfactory intercourse is taking place and that ejaculation is taking place within the vagina. Previous surgery to the cervix, diathermy or cone biopsy may be relevant.

A history of loss of ejaculate from the vagina following intercourse may be relevant.

Previous pelvic infection or chronic pelvic pain may suggest tubal damage. Dysmenorrhoea suggestive of endometriosis may be associated with tubal distortion due to intraperitoneal adhesions. Surgery such as termination of pregnancy or appendicectomy with peritonitis may have resulted in tubal damage. Tubal surgery, particularly following an ectopic pregnancy will result in subfertility as may tubal infection which may follow the use of an intrauterine contraceptive device (IUCD).

*Examination*

The presence of scars from previous surgery and any abdominal tenderness should be noted. Vaginal examination is usually normal but may reveal a fixed retroverted uterus suggestive of chronic infection or endometriosis. A distorted cervix may exist as a result of previous treatment.

*Investigation*

Cervical mucus and sperm hostility can be assessed by a postcoital test. Intercourse should take place in mid-cycle following three days without ejaculation, and a sample of cervical mucus and secretions from the posterior vaginal fornix should be examined microscopically within six hours. The cervical mucus is examined for *spinbarkeit* which is the length to which it can be stretched. The presence of sperms is noted and recorded as the number seen per high power field together with a measure of their motility. A normal test is reassuring whilst the absence of sperms may indicate that ejaculate is being lost from the vagina. The presence of a high proportion of immotile sperms may indicate that anti-sperm antibodies are present. An unsatisfactory test should be repeated and if still abnormal a crossed hostility test should be performed to establish whether the cervical mucus is impeding fertility. In this test donor sperms and mucus are paired with those of the couple to assess sperm hostility.

   Tubal patency may be assessed by laparoscopy, hystero-salpingography or the more recently introduced falloposcopy (visualization of the fallopian tubes through a telescope introduced via the cervical canal). Laparoscopy has the advantage that the inside of the pelvis can be assessed for adhesions, tubal distortion, evidence of previous infection and endometriosis as well as tubal patency. It is, however, more invasive than hysterosalpingography and requires general anaesthesia. Radiological investigation allows assessment of the uterine cavity and may be particularly useful when a cornual blockage is suspected and tubal re-implantation is being considered.

## Management

### Male factors

In general there is little that can be done to improve semen analysis. If drugs or alcohol are implicated in poor sperm production then withdrawal can lead to a dramatic improvement. Steroid therapy has been tried for poor sperm counts with limited success. Surgery may be appropriate where blockage has occurred for whatever reason but even when patency is achieved, anti-sperm antibodies may affect fertility. After vasectomy, reversal procedures may achieve up to 50% success if performed within the first five years, but only 10% after five years. If attempts to relieve a blockage are unsuccessful it may be possible to aspirate sperm from the testis for artificial insemination.

*In vitro* fertilization (IVF) is a major breakthrough in the treatment of subfertility due to male problems and may employ donor sperm or the husband's sperm. Where quality of sperm is poor as well as a low count, subzonal sperm implantation (SUZI) may be employed.

### DISCO

Direct injection of sperm into the cytoplasm of the oöcyte (DISCO) is a technique sometimes used where SUZI has failed.

Directly depositing the sperm into the cytoplasm of the egg bypasses all the natural barriers that the sperm has to encounter. On successful fertilization of the egg, the embryo then has to be transferred into the uterus for implantation to occur.

## Female factors

### Anovulation

It may be possible to induce ovulation by adjusting one's weight. In most patients ovulation can be achieved by drugs, most commonly clomiphene citrate. This has anti-oestrogen properties and its feedback on the hypothalamic–pituitary axis stimulates the release of gonadotrophins usually resulting in ovulation. In cases of hyperprolactinaemia, Bromocriptine will usually induce ovulation. The effect of the drug may be monitored by ultrasound examination of the ovaries, assessing development of follicles, as well as monitoring the mid-secretory phase progesterone. Injections of human chorionic gonadotrophin (HCG) may stimulate ovum release when the follicles have reached a certain size.

If ovulation is not achieved within six to nine months of clomiphene therapy one should offer more intensive treatment using pure FSH or a combination of FSH and LH. Whilst hyperstimulation is a relatively uncommon problem with clomiphene therapy, this is not so with analogues and one should carefully monitor oestradiol levels and follicular development prior to giving HCG to cause release of ova. If too many follicles develop one should withhold HCG until a subsequent treatment cycle. With more complicated ovulation induction techniques and particularly with IVF one may wish to down regulate the pituitary gland with luteinizing-hormone-releasing hormone (LH-RH) prior to giving analogues in order to achieve better cycle control.

In cases where ovarian failure has occurred one may consider ovum donation to achieve IVF, but this may raise ethical problems particularly in older women.

## Transport problems

Where there appears to be loss of ejaculate from the vagina, or where there are mucus problems or sperm hostility, it may be appropriate to employ artificial insemination by husband (AIH). Fresh semen specimens are injected into the cervical canal or endometrial cavity in mid-cycle for up to six cycles. Failure to achieve a pregnancy after this may be an indication for artificial insemination by donor (AID) or assisted conception techniques employing *in vivo* fertilization (gamete intrafallopian transfer – GIFT) or *in vitro* fertilization. The use of steroids or wearing a condom during intercourse for six months have been tried with dubious success to counteract anti-sperm antibodies.

GIFT is only suitable for patients who have healthy patent tubes. Oöcytes are recovered at laparoscopy, mixed with the partner's sperm and the mixture is then injected into the fallopian tube. This technique differs from IVF in that fertilization does not take place in the laboratory as it does in IVF.

## Zygote intrafallopian transfer (ZIFT)

In this technique the zygote (fertilized egg) is transferred to the fallopian tube, providing a 'natural' environment for the zygote to mature into an embryo by the time it reaches the uterus.

Tubal surgery may be indicated for either tubal blockage or peritubal adhesions. The chances of achieving a pregnancy following this will depend upon the type of surgery that has been performed. The best outlook is where the tubes are patent but adhesions require freeing. Tubal re-anastomosis following excision of a blocked segment carries a less favourable prognosis, whilst tubal re-implantation into the uterine cornua is least likely to succeed. In such circumstances resources may be better employed by carrying out three cycles of *in vitro* fertilization. The concern following tubal surgery is that a damaged tube is usually left behind in which an ectopic pregnancy is more likely to occur. The advantage of tubal surgery over *in vitro* fertilization is that if the procedure is successful once then it may be successful for subsequent pregnancies, requiring no further investigation.

### Assisted conception

In some couples one may find no cause for subfertility following extensive investigation and yet they remain unable to conceive spontaneously. In such couples assisted conception may be desired.

In IVF, fertilization occurs outside the body and the conceptus is then replaced in the uterine cavity. *In vivo* techniques such as GIFT, require normal tubes as the egg and sperm are mixed outside the body and then replaced in the tube either at laparoscopy or by falloposcopy, where it is hoped that fertilization will occur.

If an ongoing intrauterine pregnancy is not achieved after three cycles of therapy, the success rate declines rapidly and it may be more appropriate to pursue other avenues such as adoption.

### Question

**Q**: Who is suitable for egg donation to infertile couples?
**A**: The donor should usually be:
- between the ages of 18 and 35 years;
- have had healthy children and completed their family;
- be screened for HIV and hepatitis;
- not have a history of hereditary disease.

The volunteer usually receives fertility-enhancing drugs before the eggs are removed laparoscopically.

# 4: The Menopause and Premenstrual Syndrome

## The menopause

The menopause is defined as the cessation of menstruation and occurs, on average, between 50 and 52 years of age. Twenty years ago the average age was 48 years. The menopause is the combination of complex endocrine changes in which the ovaries become increasingly resistant to gonadotrophins. The first alterations in gonadotrophin response may occur 15 years prior to the menopause and 'menopausal symptoms' may become apparent long before the cessation of periods.

The first biochemical change occurring at the menopause is an increase in follicle-stimulating hormone (FSH) as a result of increased resistance of the ovaries to follicular development. Following this, the development of the corpus luteum becomes erratic with deficient progesterone secretion. Anovulatory cycles become much more common with failure of follicular development and there is a fall in oestrogen production. Finally the secretion of both FSH and luteinizing hormone (LH) increase and periods no longer occur. After this there is an increase in ovarian androgen production.

There are effects on many different organ systems and there are a multitude of symptoms that may be related to the endocrine changes associated with the menopause. It is, however, very easy to blame the menopause for a lot of problems which may present around this time, and hormone replacement therapy (HRT) may not always be appropriate therapy.

It is not surprising that because of all the complex endocrine changes occurring, many women experience abnormal vaginal bleeding in the years leading up to the menopause. Cycles often become irregular with periods becoming unpredictable and intermenstrual loss more frequent. The majority of women experiencing such problems have no underlying pathological cause but it is always important to remember that there is a gradual increase in the incidence of endometrial carcinoma from the age of 40 years onwards. It is therefore mandatory that all such women undergo a diagnostic evaluation of their endometrium before embarking upon medical therapy to manipulate their cycles.

Many other symptoms may be experienced around the time of the menopause unrelated to vaginal blood loss. No symptoms may be experienced at all by some women although they do become increasingly at risk of some diseases as a consequence of falling circulating oestrogen. Despite much research and an increased understanding of the complex changes occurring around the menopause, a number of factors including personal prejudice of the doctor, the patient's past medical history and family history and whether the patient still has a uterus or not, will all influence the decision whether to prescribe HRT or not.

### Symptoms

#### Vasomotor problems

Perhaps the commonest menopausal complaint is of hot flushes, which can occur at any time but tend to be most troublesome at night. They do not usually last long when they occur but they do cause sweating and may be associated with a tachycardia and palpitations. They usually respond dramatically to oestrogen therapy although other treatments including clonidine may be effective.

#### Genito-urinary symptoms

These are largely related to oestrogen deficiency resulting in epithelial changes in the lower genital tract. Atrophic vaginitis occurs due to the effect of lack of oestrogen on vaginal epithelium, leading to vaginal dryness and dyspareunia.

Frequency and urgency of micturition may result from atrophic changes in the lower urinary tract. Oestrogen replacement therapy is usually effective and may be administered locally rather than systemically. Vaginal lubricants including KY jelly or Replens may be useful.

## Psychological symptoms

Headaches, irritability, anxiety, loss of memory, poor concentration and failing self-esteem may all occur around the time of the menopause and are more difficult to relate to oestrogen deficiency than vasomotor and urinary symptoms. An increasing awareness of the end of the reproductive career and visible signs of ageing may contribute to these symptoms. Progesterone replacement may be appropriate although symptomatic treatment with antidepressants or psychotherapy should not be overlooked.

## Long-term consequences of oestrogen deficiency

Apart from symptomatic problems, which may last for up to a few years, longer term problems and potential risks should be considered when contemplating active intervention, particularly in women undergoing an early menopause for whatever reason.

## Osteoporosis

Oestrogen protects against bone loss and the inevitable development of osteoporosis.

Osteoporosis jeopardizes the quality of life for many postmenopausal women. It produces significant morbidity and causes significant mortality in elderly women. A woman of 50 years of age living in the West has a 15% risk of sustaining a hip fracture and a similar risk of sustaining a Colles' fracture in the remainder of her life compared with only a 5% risk in men of the same age. Other fractures, including vertebral fractures, resulting sometimes in a marked loss of height and deformity, are also more common with ageing. Whilst osteoporosis is not the only risk factor for fractures, there is such an increased risk in women after the menopause, compared with men, that prevention and treatment of osteoporosis in women can significantly improve both quality and quantity of life.

After the menopause, the reduction in oestrogen is the single most important factor resulting in loss of total or peak bone mass. Genetic and environmental factors also affect peak bone mass; black people generally have a greater bone density and therefore fewer hip fractures than the white population.

The mode of action of oestrogen in bone formation is not clearly understood but bone remodelling slows down after the menopause, as a result of the fall in circulating oestrogen. After the menopause, oestrogen levels, derived from adipose tissue, are maintained higher, therefore resulting in less osteoporosis in more obese women.

Drug treatment, in particular the use of HRT around the time of the menopause has been shown not only to slow down loss of bone resulting in osteoporosis, but also to decrease the risk of premature death due to ischaemic heart disease.

## Cardiovascular disease

The incidence of coronary heart disease in men under the age of 50 years is considerably greater than in women of the same age and this has been attributed to the protective effect of oestrogen. Following the menopause the incidence rapidly equalizes between the two sexes. The use of oestrogen replacement therapy maintains the protective effect in older women and this has major epidemiological implications, as coronary heart disease is one of the major causes of morbidity and mortality in the elderly population. There is some question as to whether the addition of progesterone in combined HRT negates the protective effect of oestrogen against cardiovascular disease.

## Disadvantages and contraindications to HRT

*Endometrial carcinoma.* The use of unopposed oestrogen has a proliferative effect upon the endometrium which will eventually cause atypical cellular changes followed by malignancy. It has been demonstrated that the addition of progesterone for 12 days of every 28-day cycle will protect the endometrium against proliferation and malignancy.

In patients who have undergone a hysterectomy this is not an issue when considering HRT.

*Breast carcinoma.* Because some breast tumours appear oestrogen dependant, there is concern over the use of oestrogen replacement and the risk of breast cancer. There is no proven increased risk of breast cancer in women taking HRT for less than 10 years. There is a suggestion of a slightly increased risk in women taking HRT for longer than this although the risk is outweighed by the protective effect against cardiovascular disease and osteoporosis.

*Other malignancies.* There does not appear to be any association between the use of HRT and other malignancies.

*Contraindications.* Contraindications against HRT have been extrapolated from the contraindications to the combined oral contraceptive pill. However, HRT involves replacement with natural hormone and does not appear to be associated with the same problems as the combined pill. There do not therefore appear to be any absolute contraindications to HRT, and particularly in patients with severe symptoms, treatment should not be withheld.

Relative contraindications include a history of breast or endometrial carcinoma, thrombo-embolic disease (although there is no evidence that any form of HRT increases the risk of thrombosis) and uncontrolled hypertension (which should be treated prior to commencing HRT).

This demonstrates the importance of treating each case on its own merits and individualizing treatment as much as possible.

### What type of HRT?

In patients without a uterus, unopposed oestrogen therapy is the treatment of choice. This can be taken orally, transdermally or by subcutaneous implant. Oestrogen given orally passes through the liver prior to systemic absorption and is partly metabolized. This is only a problem in patients with liver disease. Oral administration does not appear to have the metabolic effect of increasing bone mass which other methods of absorption do. Skin patches are well tolerated, apart from occasional skin irritation, and do give a fairly constant level of oestrogen in the circulation. Subcutaneous implants have the advantage of only having to be administered two or three times a year. However, one may get fluctuating oestrogen levels in the circulation, and the patient may become tolerant to them requiring further implants with increasing frequency. Serum oestradiol levels may become very high.

Dosage can be assessed by symptom relief and measurement of serum oestradiol levels. From the point of view of cost, oral therapy is the cheapest.

In patients who still have a uterus, progesterone must be given for 12 out of every 28 days, and this is available in tablet or patch form. Most women will have a monthly withdrawal bleed and this may deter some women from embarking upon or continuing with HRT. *Tridestra*, a new sequential combined HRT provides a quarterly bleed at the end of each three month cycle. Designed for the postmenopausal woman, it reduces the risk of osteoporosis whilst giving rise to periods only every 13 weeks. Periods are unlikely to be any heavier than normal, and 86% of women were still taking Tridestra at the end of the first year. The presentation and packaging of Tridestra is user-friendly, with 91 tablets in three blister packs, 70 tablets containing oestradiol valerate USP 2mg; 14 tablets containing oestradiol valerate USP and medroxyprogesterone acetate BP and seven placebo tablets.

An alternative treatment for women with a uterus who want HRT but do not want a withdrawal bleed, is the use of tibolone (Livial) which has androgenic properties and causes symptomatic relief, as well as being reasonably effective in preventing loss of bone density, although it is not yet licensed for this indication. Irregular menstrual bleeding may occur if tibolone is administered within 12 months of the last natural period but otherwise a withdrawal bleed is unlikely. Any bleeding which does occur on this treatment should be investigated. Tibolone is only licensed for use after 12 months of amenorrhoea.

## Contraception and the menopause

Some form of contraception is usually recommended as necessary for at least one year after the final menstrual period if this occurs after the age of 50 years or two years after the last menstrual period if this occurs under the age of 50 years. Problems can arise however in giving advice on the continuing need for contraception after the menopause if the woman is taking the combined oral contraceptive pill or the progesterone-only pill or HRT at the time of the menopause as these may continue to give rise to 'periods' or withdrawal bleeds well after the time that ovulation has ceased.

In women taking the combined pill at the time of the menopause, whilst ovarian failure and eventual cessation still occurs, symptoms of oestrogen deficiency will be masked by the pill. Diagnosis of the menopause can be achieved by stopping the combined pill, and if amenorrhoea follows, together with symptoms of the menopause and a raised FSH on two separate occasions, this is strongly suggestive of the menopause.

In women who are taking the progesterone-only pill and still having periods at the time of the menopause, there is no need to stop the pill as progesterone does not influence FSH, therefore a raised FSH, whilst still taking the minipill is diagnostic of the menopause. If a woman who is taking the progesterone-only pill is amenorrhoeic but has a normal FSH then the amenorrhoea is pill-induced, *and is not indicative that the menopause has occurred.*

In women under the age of 50, it is best to measure the FSH on two separate occasions separated by three months if contraception is to be stopped completely on reaching the menopause and simple non-hormonal contraception used for 12 months for absolute safety.

Women reaching the menopause and taking HRT will still get a rise in FSH, despite the small dose of exogenous oestrogen but this is a less reliable indicator of being able to stop using some form of contraception.

Barrier methods may be less acceptable as an alternative method of contraception, around the time of the menopause, due either to vaginal dryness or erectile dysfunction.

The intrauterine contraceptive device (IUCD) may be a very acceptable form of contraception for the older woman and any device fitted after the age of 40 years can probably be left *in situ* until one year after the menopause or until age 53 years if the woman is taking HRT.

Sterilization, by one or other partner has often been chosen as a method before the menopause has been reached.

Low dose combined contraceptive pills or progesterone-only pills are acceptable and safe up to the menopause provided that no contraindications to either exist.

## Premenstrual syndrome

Premenstrual Syndrome (PMS) is still poorly defined and understood despite considerable research. The aetiology is probably multifactorial. Hormonal alterations appear to be of importance, but psychogenic and social factors also contribute to the syndrome. Ovulation is a prerequisite to the development of PMS and some treatments are aimed at its suppression. The clinical presentation is varied and results in a mixture of physical and psychogenic symptoms. Other conditions, particularly psychiatric disorders, may be confused with PMS and a positive diagnosis is dependent upon the cyclical nature of the patient's symptoms. These tend to occur premenstrually but may persist throughout and even following menstruation.

## Aetiology

The following have been suggested:
1 decreased luteal phase progesterone;
2 increased circulating oestrogen;
3 raised oestrogen : progesterone ratio;
4 decreased levels of vitamin $B_6$ and vitamin A;
5 Psychogenic factors.

## Symptoms

The symptomatology may be physical or psychological, but is usually a mixture of the two.

*Physical symptoms*
- Fluid retention causing breast discomfort and abdominal distension
- Abdominal pain
- Back pain
- Muscular aches and pains
- Headache
- Nausea and vomiting
- Dizziness
- Sweating
- Palpitations

*Psychological symptoms*
- Anxiety
- Depression

- Labile mood
- Lethargy
- Impaired performance
- Poor concentration
- Behavioural disturbance

## Treatment

A variety of different therapies have been tried based upon the varied aetiological theories. Unfortunately the results in double-blind trials have often been disappointing. No individual treatment regimen provides consistently successful results but the following have all been used.

*Non-hormonal treatments*
- Oil of evening primrose
- Vitamin $B_6$
- High carbohydrate diet
- Lithium
- Antidepressants

*Hormonal treatments*
- Cyclical progestogens
- Oral contraceptive pill
- HRT
- Danazol
- Pregnancy

*Surgical treatments*
- bilateral oöphorectomy (possibly combined with hysterectomy).

A sensible initial approach is to recommend oil of evening primrose or vitamin $B_6$ together with a proportionally increased carbohydrate intake, for a period of at least three, preferably six months. If these measures are not beneficial, the combined oral contraceptive pill or HRT may be effective. Cyclical progestogens are probably less successful but suppositories may be more useful, though less acceptable to the patient, than oral preparations.

Pregnancy usually eradicates any symptoms of PMS.

In very severe and unresponsive cases of PMS, oöphorectomy, combined with hysterectomy, should be considered. Hysterectomy alone is unlikely to be beneficial.

## Questions

**Q1**: Which investigations should be performed before and during prescribing HRT?

**A**: Perimenopausal women who are having menopausal type symptoms, but are still menstruating, are likely to have failing ovarian function resulting in low levels of serum oestradiol, 100–200 pmol/l, and a high FSH, >15–20 pmol/l, occasionally >30 pmol/l. Other investigations are unnecessary. It is sensible to check blood pressure and examine the breasts annually.

Serum oestradiol levels may be worth considering in patients who fail to respond to therapeutic doses of oestrogen. A low measured level will indicate poor compliance or poor absorption, whereas a normal level indicates that the symptoms are not due to the effect of the menopause. Plasma oestradiol levels should be checked annually in women having implants.

**Q2**: What sort of HRT, if any, can I prescribe for a patient with known fibroids?

**A**: Fibroids are not a contraindication to the use of HRT at the time of the menopause but oestrogen may cause them to grow. Likewise fibroids often shrink after the menopause due to lack of oestrogen stimulus. Whether oestrogen should be used at all to treat symptoms associated with the menopause depends upon the size of the fibroids and the presence of any

other pathology such as ovarian pathology and/or endometrial hyperplasia.

Vaginal ultrasound examination may be useful to deter-
mine whether either of these pathologies is present.

With regard to which HRT is preferable, tibolone (Livial)
has least oestrogen-stimulating effect and would therefore be
an ideal choice in a woman who is more than a year post-
menopause.

**Q3**: Is it acceptable to prescribe HRT to hypertensive women?
**A**: Yes. Hypertension may be an indication rather than a
contraindication to prescribing HRT, according to the British
Menopause Society. The cardiovascular benefits of HRT out-
weigh the risk, if any, of prescribing HRT to someone whose
blood pressure is adequately controlled. Therefore, before
commencing HRT, raised blood pressure should be dealt with
in the usual way and once satisfactory control is acheived,
HRT may be prescribed.

**Q4**: Can women with a past history of deep venous thrombosis
(DVT) be given HRT?
**A**: Yes. There is no evidence that HRT increases the risk of
thrombosis although transdermal delivery is theoretically
safer because of its lack of effect on hepatic clotting factors.

**Q5**: Are there any medical advantages in favouring one route of
administration (e.g. transdermal) to another (e.g. oral or
implant)?
**A**: Most of the evidence accumulated so far from the cardio-
protective effect of HRT is based on oral preparations though
there is no reason to suspect that other delivery systems are
less good. Transdermal therapy does however have a beneficial effect upon serum triglycerides whereas some oral therapies can raise triglycerides. Transdermal therapy is also
theoretically favoured in women with a past history of DVT

although there is no evidence of any increased risk of DVT with any form of HRT.

Oral oestradiol however may be preferable in women at risk of heart disease who have low high-density lipoproteins because these are increased more by oral therapy than by the transdermal route.

**Q6**: Does HRT reduce blood loss in perimenopausal women?

**A**: HRT may be helpful in reducing blood loss at the menopause though it is probably less effective than other options and of course should only be considered when pathology has been excluded.

**Q7**: How long should HRT be prescribed?

**A**: Epidemiologically it would be logical to prescribe HRT to all women indefinitely. However, other factors must be considered such as symptomatology, the need for a monthly withdrawal bleed, the presence of relative contraindications, the presence of progestogenic side-effects (fluid retention, bloating and abdominal discomfort) and the woman's own anxiety about taking long-term medication.

Women going through the menopause under the age of 50 years should be encouraged to take HRT, at least until the average age of the menopause. HRT should be discussed with, and where appropriate made readily available to, all menopausal women. This role is increasingly being placed upon general practitioners and their practice nurses.

# 5: Gynaecological Emergencies

Gynaecological emergencies are common and are therefore frequently presented in primary care. They can be classified as emergencies related to pregnancy or emergencies not related to pregnancy. Most gynaecological emergencies associated with pregnancy can be life-threatening, for mother or fetus, and some emergencies not related to pregnancy can also be life-threatening.

Some gynaecological emergencies, occurring during pregnancy, can also occur in the non-pregnant state and they therefore will be considered under the non-pregnancy related conditions.

**Pregnancy related emergencies**

Complications of pregnancy may be related to intrauterine or extrauterine gestation.

*Intrauterine complications of pregnancy*

Abortion may be any one of the following types.
1 Threatened.
2 Inevitable.
3 Incomplete.
4 Complete.
5 Missed.
6 Septic.
7 Therapeutic.

All of these, except therapeutic, may be considered as gynaecological emergencies although missed abortions are more often diagnosed on routine ultrasound examination.

The others present with a period of amenorrhoea, most often

40

in the first 12 weeks of pregnancy, and are associated with abnormal bleeding and varying degrees of lower abdominal pain. The bleeding is usually fresh and heavy and there may be blood clots. The pain is usually suprapubic and cramp-like and similar to a severe 'period pain'. The patient has frequently had a positive pregnancy test and may have associated symptoms of pregnancy including nausea, sometimes accompanied by vomiting, increased frequency of micturition and breast tenderness.

The type or stage of the abortion may be determined by clinical examination although ultrasound examination is invaluable and sometimes mandatory in confirming viability of the fetus. In primary care, miscarriage or threatened miscarriage often occurs at the patient's home and a bimanual vaginal examination is not always easy or practical, though it can provide useful information about the state of the cervix.

Abdominal examination is often unhelpful, although the uterus should be palpable if the gestation is greater than 12 weeks, and marked abdominal tenderness may be suggestive of other diagnoses such as ectopic pregnancy or pelvic inflammatory disease (PID).

On vaginal examination, the state of the cervix is important. Cervical excitation, severe tenderness on moving the cervix laterally, may be suggestive of an ectopic pregnancy if unilateral or salpingitis if bilateral. Cervical excitation pain is caused by stretching the peritoneum overlying the fallopian tube on the affected side, with the uterine body acting as a fulcrum.

The cervix is closed in threatened miscarriage, but opens to allow the uterus to expel the products of conception in inevitable and incomplete abortions. When the abortion is complete the cervix closes again. Whilst the cervix is open it is possible to pass one or even two fingers into the uterine cavity without difficulty and at this stage non-viability of the gestation is confirmed. In all other situations an ultrasound examination of the pelvis and uterine contents will clarify the situation and confirm or refute viability.

If the uterine size on clinical or ultrasound examination is smaller than the history suggests, this may indicate a missed, incomplete or complete abortion, or possibly an ectopic pregnancy (see below). When a patient gives a history of a complete abortion, at less than six weeks gestation, she can often be managed at home without hospital intervention, although anti-D immunization may be required (see below). A history of complete abortion, at home, in patients greater than 12 weeks gestation almost invariably require hospitalization and a dilatation and curettage (D&C).

If a viable intrauterine pregnancy is confirmed, bed rest should be recommended until the bleeding subsides. Hospital admission should be considered if the bleeding is heavy or persistent or accompanied by moderately severe pain, or if social circumstances dictate.

If the gestation is confirmed on ultrasound to be non-viable, evacuation of the uterus should be performed unless a complete abortion has occurred and the bleeding has settled.

*Anti-D immunoglobulin should be given following evacuation of the uterus in rhesus-negative women, although the need for immunoglobulin in early threatened or complete miscarriage is not conclusively proven.*

Miscarriage is extremely common and patients can generally be reassured that a single miscarriage is unlikely to adversely affect the chances of a subsequent successful pregnancy. Nevertheless miscarriage can cause significant distress and support should be available and offered to all women.

Since therapeutic abortion has been legalized, the incidence of septic abortion has declined considerably. When it does occur it is most common after therapeutic abortion has been performed but without complete evacuation of the uterus.

The presention of *septic abortion* usually includes generalized signs and symptoms of infection, sometimes septicaemia, associated with severe lower abdominal pain and vaginal bleeding. Whether the cervix is open or closed will indicate the presence or absence of retained products. Antibiotics are essential and the patient will usually require hospitalization.

Pelvic ultrasound is not usually necessary or helpful. If the cervical os is open, a careful uterine curettage by an experienced gynaecologist after 24 hours of antibiotics should reduce the high risk of uterine perforation. If vaginal bleeding is heavy, curettage may need to be carried out without the preceding 24-hour antibiotic cover; intravenous antibiotics may be substituted. If the cervix appears closed but the patient's general condition does not improve within 48 hours, curettage may then be necessary.

*The management of bleeding following therapeutic abortion, outlined above, is the same as secondary postpartum haemorrhage following childbirth.*

### Extrauterine complications of pregnancy

*Ectopic pregnancy*

Ectopic pregnancy is the most dangerous gynaecological emergency. Its presentation can vary from a shocked moribund woman following a catastrophic intraperitoneal haemorrhage, to an asymptomatic patient with a positive pregnancy test and an empty uterine cavity on ultrasound scan.

Because of the potentially serious nature, all patients presenting as a gynaecological emergency should have ectopic pregnancy excluded as a priority.

The majority of ectopic pregnancies occur in the fallopian tubes, but other sites include the ovary, cervix and peritoneal cavity (abdominal pregnancy).

Risk factors for ectopic pregnancy include any condition resulting in intrinsic tubal damage or tubal distortion such as pelvic infection, tubal surgery or other intraperitoneal surgery. Conception with a coil *in situ* should raise the possibility of an ectopic pregnancy. Ectopic pregnancy rate is *not* increased in coil users, but because the coil protects against intrauterine pregnancy only, the actual number of ectopic pregnancies will be relatively greater in coil users than in non-coil users.

There is also an increased risk of ectopic pregnancy in women undergoing assisted-conception techniques, particularly those involving patent tubes such as gamete intrafallopian transfer (GIFT). *Ectopic pregnancy occurring in combination with intrauterine pregnancy is extremely rare with an incidence of about 1 in 30000 conceptions.*

Ectopic pregnancies usually present earlier than threatened miscarriage and the three main symptoms are:
• a short period of amenorrhoea;
• unilateral lower abdominal pain;
• abnormal vaginal bleeding.

These symptoms also can occur in threatened abortion and the differentiation can be extremely difficult.

The period of amenorrhoea in ectopic pregnancy is often about six weeks although the patient may not describe missing a period at all but rather that the last period was different from previous ones.

The bleeding associated with ectopic pregnancy is often much less heavy than with abortion and is characteristically much darker in colour (sometimes described as like 'prune juice').

Abdominal examination may reveal unilateral tenderness although this may be more generalized if there has been any intraperitoneal bleeding. Vaginal examination may cause unilateral cervical excitation as the peritoneum over the gestation sac is stretched. It is rare to feel a mass with ectopic pregnancy and if one is felt it should raise the question of a possible ovarian cyst.

If the history is suggestive of an ectopic pregnancy and there is cervical excitation present on pelvic examination, extreme care must be taken to avoid possible rupture of the gestation sac and if the patient is not already in hospital she should be sent there immediately.

As well as threatened abortion, the other differential diagnosis is pelvic infection, acute salpingitis. A history of bilateral lower abdominal/pelvic pain accompanied by a smelly vaginal discharge and a fever would suggest possible pelvic infection as may a past history of previous episodes of similar presenting symptoms. *A raised temperature may occur in ectopic pregnancy if there has been intraperitoneal bleeding* although this virtually never exceeds 38°C.

## Investigations

These may be unhelpful in ectopic pregnancy.

A full blood count may show anaemia.

Modern urinary pregnancy tests measuring beta-human chorionic gonadotrophin (HCG) are extremely sensitive and will usually be positive in ectopic pregnancy. Serum beta-HCG tests are even more sensitive.

Pelvic ultrasound scanning will not usually show an ectopic pregnancy although the use of the *vaginal ultrasound probe* greatly increases the sensitivity of the procedure (fewer false negatives).

The situation may then arise of a positive pregnancy test and an empty uterine cavity on ultrasound scan. The differential diagnosis will be an ectopic pregnancy and an early intrauterine pregnancy and the management will be dependent upon clinical judgement. It may be necessary to investigate further with laparoscopy, to confirm or refute the diagnosis of ectopic pregnancy or it may be appropriate to measure serial beta-HCGs which increase more rapidly in intrauterine pregnancy than in ectopic pregnancy. *Whilst the diagnosis of an ectopic pregnancy is under consideration the patient should always be in hospital.*

## Management of ectopic pregnancy

This is by the removal of the pregnancy which may be performed laparoscopically or by laparotomy. The method will be determined by the clinical situation which in turn will depend upon the size, gestation and amount of bleeding. There is an increasing tendency towards performing the removal of the pregnancy with tubal preservation, particularly in small unruptured gestations, although this will clearly *increase the subsequent risk of further tubal pregnancy* which would not occur if salpingectomy was performed.

Cervical pregnancy usually presents as an inevitable abortion and only becomes apparent when there is difficulty stopping bleeding at the time of evacuation of the uterus. In these circumstances a hysterectomy may become necessary occasionally.

*Fertility* is considerably reduced following ectopic pregnancy and the risk of further ectopic pregnancy is greatly increased. *Less than 50% of women will ever give birth to a live child after an ectopic pregnancy.*

## Non-pregnancy related emergencies

### *Ovaries*

Ovarian cysts can undergo the following complications.
1 Rupture.
2 Haemorrhage.
3 Torsion.
4 Infection.
5 Malignant change.

All except malignant change may present as an emergency. NB Luteal cysts can undergo changes and complications in association with pregnancy and it should also be remembered that such cysts may disappear spontaneously as pregnancy advances.

*Rupture and bleeding* from ovarian cysts usually present as sudden onset abdominal pain, often severe and maximal in the lower abdomen but there may quickly develop generalized pain with peritoneal irritation. The patient may quickly become shocked, particularly if there is heavy bleeding. Examination may reveal signs of localized or generalized peritonitis, with marked tenderness and guarding. A mass may not be obviously palpable particularly if the cyst has collapsed. There may be extreme tenderness on vaginal and rectal examination.

The diagnosis may be difficult to distinguish from ruptured ectopic pregnancy and an immediate laparotomy may be necessary to distinguish between the two and treat appropriately.

Lesser degrees of bleeding or rupture of a small locule of a cyst may present less dramatically and a cyst may even be palpated on abdominal or vaginal examination. The diagnosis of an ovarian cyst can be confirmed with a pelvic ultrasound examination. Laparoscopic assessment with aspiration or open cystectomy may become necessary.

*Torsion* of an ovarian cyst usually presents with acute pain which is colicky in nature. There is often a history of previous episodes of a similar pain. Ultrasound examination will confirm the presence of a cyst which should be treated surgically at laparotomy. If the ovary is gangrenous it must be removed but otherwise ovarian cystectomy with fixation of the remaining portion of the ovary is undertaken. Usually it is prudent to fix the other ovary at the same time by suturing it to the pelvic side wall.

*Ovarian abscesses* may arise *de novo* or occur in conjunction with acute salpingitis. There is usually an acute febrile illness with lower abdominal pain and signs of local peritonitis. Extreme tenderness may be elicited on vaginal examination. Unless there is generalized peritonitis suggested by leakage of pus, the patient should be managed conservatively initially with intravenous fluids, antibiotics and analgesics. The patient's general condition should be monitored carefully over 48 hours with an assessment of the size of the abscess carried out using a pelvic ultrasound examination. If there is clinical improvement, with decreasing size on pelvic ultrasound, conservative management should be maintained; otherwise laparotomy with drainage and possible oöphorectomy may need to be under-taken. In patients with bilateral abscesses who have completed their families it may be appropriate to clear the pelvis with a hysterectomy and bilateral salpingo-oöphorectomy. This procedure, though less desirable, is sometimes necessary in younger women. The pelvis should be drained postoperatively with continuing antibiotic treatment.

## *Fallopian tubes*

Acute PID most commonly affects the fallopian tubes and the subject is considered in detail in Chapter 8 on Pelvic Infection.

## *Uterus*

*Dysfunctional uterine bleeding (DUB)* can present with extremely heavy vaginal bleeding occasionally necessitating urgent hospital admission. It is commonest in women over the age of 40 years and there is usually a preceding history of menstrual dysfunction and possibly known fibroids.

The patient may be shocked and the emergency can be con-fused with threatened abortion. A sensitive pregnancy test will help to eliminate this from the differential diagnosis.

Progestogens or oestrogens may be sufficient to control the bleeding but if necessary, due to very heavy bleeding, an emer-gency curettage will always stop the bleeding.

In the postmenopausal woman, an endometrial carcinoma may occasionally present with heavy vaginal bleeding, necessi-tating hospital admission though rarely necessitating emer-gency curettage.

## *Cervix*

Cervical malignancy may occasionally present with heavy vaginal bleeding, more commonly seen in more advanced disease. It may be one of the few indications for emergency radiotherapy.

Following *cone biopsy* of the cervix, secondary haemorrhage requiring admission to hospital and suturing may be necessary in up to 10% of patients.

## Vagina

Bleeding from the vagina may occur following trauma. This is usually in young women following their first attempt at intercourse; or in postmenopausal women, again following intercourse, bleeding occurring from atrophic tissues. It is usually necessary to suture traumatic tears under anaesthetic.

Vaginal bleeding may also present as an emergency following hysterectomy and repair procedures. It is often possible to manage conservatively, in these circumstances, particularly following drainage of a vault haematoma, although occasionally suturing may be required.

## Vulva

Vulval abscesses particularly those of the Bartholin's glands are relatively common and usually present as a painful tender swelling of the labia. They are sometimes treated in primary care with a broad spectrum antibiotic but usually require surgical drainage in order to prevent recurrence. In addition, where possible Bartholin's abscesses are less likely to recur if they are marsupialized.

*Vulval trauma* may result in tears causing bleeding, as in the vagina, or in the occurrence of vulval haematomas. If a vulval haematoma presents within 24 hours it should be drained surgically, but after 24 hours it usually solidifies and it then becomes necessary to await resorption of the haematoma. Vulval carcinomas rarely present with heavy bleeding (see Chapter 9, Common Gynaecological Malignancies).

## Question

**Q**: When and what investigations are appropriate following miscarriage?

**A**: Cytogenetic study of the parents may be helpful and appropriate if the aborted fetus is known or suspected of having a chromosomal defect, or where a mother has three or more consecutive miscarriages. Autosomal translocation carries a 12% risk of an abnormality with a female carrier and a 5% risk with a male carrier. In such pregnancies amniocentesis is advisable.

If chromosome analysis is required, buccal smears or blood samples are taken and the result may take up to two months.

# 6: Pelvic Pain and Endometriosis

Pelvic pain is a common problem, and may be caused by numerous conditions both gynaecological and non-gynaecological. Most gynaecological causes of pelvic pain are considered elsewhere in the text. Ovarian cysts, ectopic pregnancy, abortion and acute pelvic infection are discussed in Chapter 5 on Gynaecological Emergencies whilst chronic infection is considered in Chapter 8 on Pelvic Infection.

Painful periods (dysmenorrhoea) is one of the most common gynaecological complaints, in the UK approximately 13 women per 1000 population consult their general practitioner each year because of dysmenorrhoea. A woman who has always suffered from painful periods has primary dysmenorrhoea which is rarely associated with pathology. Secondary dysmenorrhoea however after years of painless periods is more likely to be due to pathology such as endometriosis, fibroids, polyps, adenomyosis or pelvic inflammatory disease (PID).

Endometriosis may be suggested by pain (during, before and even after the period), menorrhagia, vaginal discharge, infertility and dyspareunia, both superficial and deep.

This chapter will also deal with non-gynaecological causes of pelvic pain.

## Endometriosis

This is a condition in which endometrium appears in a variety of ectopic sites giving rise to symptoms and problems related to their location. There are two theories of the origin of endometriosis. The first theory involves retrograde passage of endometrium through the tubes with implantation in the pelvis. The second theory is of spontaneous development of endometrium from totipotent cells within the peritoneal

cavity. As with uterine endometrium, this ectopic endometrium is dependant upon ovarian function to fuel it and the
mainstay of medical treatment is ovarian suppression inducing
a 'temporary menopausal state'.

Endometriosis is a relatively common condition and is said
to occur more frequently in middle class nulliparous women. In
many women the presence of endometriosis does not cause
symptoms though it may present in a number of ways.

## Symptoms

*Painful heavy periods.* Severe pain may be experienced around
the time of a period, caused by bleeding from the ectopic
endometrium resulting in peritoneal irritation. Adenomyosis
(ectopic endometrium within the myometrium) may cause
severe cramp-like pain associated with heavy bleeding.

*Chronic pelvic pain.* In the more advanced disease the pain
may become continuous due to possible pelvic adhesions and
ovarian masses or cysts.

*Dyspareunia.* Deep dyspareunia is quite a common symptom
in endometriosis. Deposits frequently occur in the Pouch of
Douglas and on the uterosacral ligaments, and in addition the
uterus may be retroverted and become relatively immobile.

*Pelvic mass.* Large endometriotic cysts may occur on the
ovaries giving rise to abdominal swelling and a mass arising
from the pelvis.

*Infertility.* Endometriosis is quite often associated with infertility. This can be due to anatomical distortion caused by adhesions but there may be other factors involved.

*Gastrointestinal symptoms.* These may result from external
pressure on the lower bowel but can also be caused by direct

infiltration of endometriotic deposits through the bowel serosa which can result in rectal bleeding. Infiltration of the umbilicus may result in a chronically discharging umbilicus which can only be treated by excision.

## Signs

Abdominal palpation may reveal a mass arising from the pelvis or there may be lower abdominal tenderness on palpation. Vaginal inspection may reveal endometriotic nodules on the cervix or in the Pouch of Douglas. Palpation may reveal a tender retroverted immobile uterus or an ovarian mass. Nodules may be palpable behind the cervix. One of the commonest sites of endometriosis is either of the uterosacral ligaments; and a rectal examination is an essential part of the examination in a patient suspected of having endometriosis.

Rectal and vaginal examinations may be normal in patients with minor degrees of endometriosis.

## Investigations

Pelvic *ultrasound scan* may reveal a pelvic mass.

*Laparoscopy* is the most important investigation in assessing the presence, absence or extent of the disease. Endometriotic deposits are seen as black spots or scarring associated with adhesions and fixation of organs.

## Treatment

Treatment is tailored to specific problems caused by the presence of endometriosis. A few black spots found during laparoscopy, with no obvious symptoms requires no treatment at all. The aim of treatment is to eradicate the disease and prevent its recurrence. This may be achieved by suppression of ovarian function or by surgical destruction or excision. The methods of treatment are as follows.

*Ovarian suppression with:*
- oral contraceptive pill;
- progestogens;
- danazol;
- luteinizing-hormone-releasing hormone (LH-RH) analogues;
- pregnancy.

*Surgical destruction by:*
- diathermy;
- laser.

*Surgical excision by:*
- conservative (either laparoscopic or open);
- total abdominal hysterectomy (TAH) with bilateral salpingo-oöphorectomy (BSO).

The type of treatment is determined by the problem it causes and the extent of disease. Medical treatment is usually first-line therapy in less extensive disease. The oral contraceptive pill and progestogen therapy are much cheaper and associated with fewer side-effects than danazol and LH-RH analogues. Medical treatment should be effective within six to nine months of commencement if it is going to be successful.

In very extensive disease surgical excision is usually required and it may be necessary to clear the pelvis to relieve severe pain even in relatively young women. Ovarian conservation in such women will result in only short-term suppression of the symptoms.

The timing of starting hormone replacement therapy (HRT) following pelvic clearance is controversial. Theoretically, the administration of oestrogen immediately following oöphorectomy may continue to feed the disease. This has not been conclusively shown and the majority are in favour of early commencement of such treatment.

## Dyspareunia

Dyspareunia is pain associated with intercourse and is classified as *superficial* or *deep*. This differentiation is important as the causes and therefore treatments vary considerably.

## Superficial

Superficial dyspareunia describes pain at or around the vaginal introitus which interferes with penetration. However once penetration has been achieved the pain may disappear. Causes of superficial dyspareunia are as follows.

*Anatomical.* A tight entrance due to hymenal remnants or iatrogenic post-surgical causes.

*Functional.* Vaginal dryness due to atrophic changes or generally poor vaginal lubrication.

*Pathological.* Various infections may cause superficial dyspareunia particularly candida trichomonas and herpes; also pruritus vulvae due to non-neoplastic vulval disorders or other dermatoses.

The treatments of *anatomical* causes usually commence with conservative measures such as the use of vaginal dilators. Subsequently, examination under anaesthesia with 'stretching' may be indicated or even surgical enlargement of the introitus.

*Functional* causes may be managed with local oestrogens or lubricants. In the postmenopausal women Replens may be suitable.

It is extremely common for women in the postnatal period to complain of dyspareunia and to worry that they have been 'stitched up too tight' following an episiotomy. At this time, and particularly in those who are breast feeding the level of circulating oestrogen is very low due to the antagonistic effect of prolactin and the vaginal tissues are dry and atrophic as a consequence. The situation usually corrects itself spontaneously with the resumption of ovulation.

*Pathological* causes of superficial dyspareunia will require treatment dependent upon the underlying pathology, e.g. treatment of the underlying infection or dermatoses.

### Deep

Deep dyspareunia describes pain felt deep in the pelvis or lower abdomen during intercourse. The pain may subside following intercourse or may continue for some time afterwards. It is much more commonly associated with significant disease than superficial dyspareunia, and is usually due to pressure caused by deep penetration.

Other causes of deep dyspareunia include distended bowel due to constipation or wind, a retroverted uterus, significant disease of the pelvic organs such as ovarian cysts, endometriosis, acute or chronic PID.

Unless there is an obvious physical cause on clinical examination, investigations should include diagnostic laparoscopy.

Clinical management will depend upon clinical findings including laparoscopic findings. If no cause is apparent, after appropriate investigation, advice on adopting different positions during sexual intercourse may be worthwhile as may referral for psychosexual assessment and counselling.

### Non-gynaecological causes of pelvic pain

The commonest group of non-gynaecological causes of pelvic pain arise from the gastrointestinal tract but urinary tract conditions and vascular problems may also cause pelvic pain.

*Gastrointestinal causes.* These tend to be functional rather than pathological, and the main problems are constipation or irritable bowel. A careful history relating these to the menstrual cycle may help to differentiate from other causes and a trial of laxatives or antispasmodics may be appropriate and may prevent hospital referral in dubious cases. Diverticular disease may give rise to pelvic pain in older women.

In cases where the pain is acute, appendicitis should be considered and may be difficult to manage other than by hospitalization for observation and surgery where appropriate.

*Urinary causes.* Problems such as urinary tract infections may give rise to pelvic pain which may be due to diverticulae or renal calculi. Routine urine testing for protein and blood may provide a useful clue in cases of pelvic pain of unknown origin.

*Vascular causes.* Chronic pelvic pain for which no obvious cause is found may be due to pelvic venous congestion. This may be demonstrated on venography or may be seen during laparoscopy. A variety of therapies may be tried such as analgesics, anti-inflammatory agents and hormonal treatments.

## Questions

**Q1**: What are the commonest causes of non-gynaecological chronic pelvic pain?
**A**: Irritable bowel syndrome and ilio-inguinal nerve entrapment, which most commonly arises from scar tissue following a laterally placed appendix scar or a low transverse incision for pelvic surgery. The diagnosis of ilio-inguinal nerve entrapment may be suspected from the history and can be confirmed by locating a trigger point in the abdominal wall and relieving symptoms by an injection of a local anaesthetic.

Eighty per cent of women undergoing laparoscopy for the investigation of chronic pelvic pain have no demonstrable abnormality.

Pelvic venous congestion, characterized by shifting pelvic pain exacerbated by standing, deep dyspareunia and post-coital aching, may benefit from hormonal treatment in the form of medroxyprogesterone acetate 30–50 mg daily for four to six months.

**Q2**: When should a patient with chronic pelvic pain be referred?

**A**: A patient should be referred if there are any abnormal physical signs such as a fixed retroverted uterus, or other distressing symptoms such as dyspareunia or menorrhagia, or if the patient's life is becoming disrupted as a result of the symptoms.

# 7: Disorders of the Vulva

Disorders of the vulva may be classified as:
1 non-neoplastic vulval disorder;
  (a) lichen sclerosis;
  (b) squamous hyperplasia;
2 vulval infections;
3 vulval intra-epithelial neoplasia;
4 carcinoma of the vulva;
5 other dermatoses affecting the vulva.

Infections, including human papilloma virus (HPV) and the more common sexually transmitted diseases (STDs), are dealt with in Chapter 8, Pelvic Infection.

Other dermatoses which may affect the vulva will not be dealt with further, but in any case where there is an unusual appearance or any condition which does not respond to the more usual treatments for non-neoplastic disorders, referral for a dermatological opinion and probable biopsy should be sought.

## Non-neoplastic vulval disorders

*Lichen sclerosis.* This is a common condition which may occur at any age in women though it is most often seen post-menopause. It is characterized by thinning of the epithelium with a homogeneous subepithelial layer in the dermis, and ultimately results in loss of the vulval architecture. The labia majora and minora become less well-defined and there may be changes in the appearance of the skin with *areas of cracking and small haemorrhages, and a whitish discoloration.*

*Vulval hyperplasia.* This may occur in any age group but is most common postmenopausally. It is characterized by elongation and widening of the ridges of the epidermis with an inflammatory infiltrate in the dermis.

Both lesions, lichen sclerosis and vulval hyperplasia may be associated with malignant change and the commonest symptom in both conditions of possible malignant transformation is *vulval pruritus and soreness*. In cases where there is doubt about the appearance, or suspicion of possible malignancy (cracking or haemorrhage or ulceration of the skin), referral is indicated for biopsy.

Treatment of these conditions may be difficult, the mainstay of treatment is topical steroid creams. It is usual to begin with low-dose steroid creams, starting with 1% hydrocortisone, applied as required, usually twice daily to the affected area. If this is unsuccessful after a sufficient period of time such as two weeks, then in lichen sclerosis, 1% testosterone cream may be tried. Otherwise a short course of four to six weeks of a more potent topical steroid such as Betnovate or Dermovate may be tried in either condition. These creams should not be used for any longer periods than four to six weeks because of the risk of systemic absorption.

In resistant cases, other treatments may include subdermal alcohol injections, destruction of skin using diathermy, laser vaporization or surgical excision. All of these treatments may result in severe discomfort and may only have a limited effect. Unfortunately, the skin changes often occur later in skin which has been moved over to cover areas of surgical excision.

Oestrogen creams are often tried in these conditions because the vulva appears 'atrophic'. They are virtually never of any benefit and their prescription should be avoided for conditions causing vulval pruritus.

### Vulval intra-epithelial neoplasia

Vulval intra-epithelial neoplasia (VIN) is a squamous pre-malignant lesion occurring on the vulva which is identical to cervical intra-epithelial neoplasia (CIN), occurring intra-epithelially in the cervix.

Both VIN and CIN share similar risk factors, in particular an association with infection with HPV. Vulval intra-epithelial neoplasia may be asymptomatic, detected at the time of colposcopic assessment of the cervix, or it may be detected on vulval inspection, with a whitish appearance more marked with the application of acetic acid. The colposcopic appearance of VIN is similar to CIN although vessel changes tend to be less marked in VIN because of the keratin covering the epidermis. Vulval intra-epithelial neoplasia may also present with vulval pruritus and may be unifocal or multifocal.

The management of VIN is much more difficult and controversial than CIN. Whilst approximately 50% of CIN III lesions will progress to invasive cancer if left untreated, it is thought that less than 10% of VIN III will do so. In addition the treatment of VIN is much more mutilating than CIN and is associated with significant morbidity, particularly sexual dysfunction.

If VIN is asymptomatic, an expectant approach is certainly followed with VIN I and VIN II, with regular follow-up and annual colposcopic examination. Vulval intra-epithelial neoplasia III should probably be managed in the same way unless there is a well-localized lesion that can be easily excised with minimal anatomical distortion, or there is sufficient concern that an early invasive lesion may be present, in which case a wide excisional biopsy of the appropriate area should be undertaken.

If VIN is symptomatic then it should be treated either with local destruction, after appropriate biopsy, or with diathermy or laser vaporization, or it should be excised. As with non-neoplastic disorders, there is a risk of skin changes occurring in the transposed skin and long-term follow-up is essential.

## Carcinoma of the vulva

This is a rare tumour which tends to affect elderly women. Ninety-five per cent of tumours are squamous carcinomas, with the second most common malignancy being malignant melanoma. Carcinoma of the vulva may arise in a pre-existing area of VIN and may be associated with hyperplasia or lichen sclerosis.

It may present with soreness or bleeding and discharge from a cracked and possibly ulcerated skin lesion.

The diagnosis should be confirmed by an adequate biopsy, and the recommended treatment for all squamous carcinomas except those that are only just invading through the basement membrane is radical vulvectomy. This involves removal of the whole of the vulval skin including wide excision of the tumour, and removal of the inguinal and superficial femoral lymph glands on both sides.

Except in the case of large tumours, the groin incisions are separated from the vulval margins and this aids skin healing. If the tumour is large and fixed, it may be possible to make it surgically resectable after a three-month course of radiotherapy and/or chemotherapy. These treatments are not applicable in most other cases of vulval cancer, except in palliation in advanced disease, in an attempt to avoid distressing complications such as fistulae formation.

The prognosis for small tumours with negative nodes is generally excellent, but as with all carcinomas, more advanced disease carries a much worse prognosis.

Malignant melanoma should be managed by wide local excision as in other areas of the body, and the prognosis is largely dependant upon the depth of invasion.

## Question

Q: How common is genital herpes and how should it be managed and by whom? Is genital herpes during pregnancy a cause for concern?

A: A general practitioner with a list of 2000 patients will expect to see about two new cases of genital herpes each year. Its presentation can be genuinely described as an emergency because it is so extremely painful. If the patient presents in surgery she may have difficulty in walking and difficulty in urinating. The primary attack is often said to be the worst and most painful. Primary or secondary attacks respond well to acyclovir or famciclovir, but oral analgesia may be required also. Topical treatments are probably ineffective. Consideration should be given to referral to a genito-urinary medicine department for follow-up and screening for other associated infections.

Active genital herpes at the time of delivery is considered a reason for delivery by caesarean section to avoid infection reaching the neonate. A primary attack of genital herpes during pregnancy can affect the fetus and close consultation with the consultant obstetrician is essential.

# 8: Pelvic Infection

Symptoms of pelvic infection are commonly presented to the general practitioner and symptoms unresponsive to treatment are a common cause of referral to gynaecology out-patient clinics. Pelvic infection may be caused by a wide variety of different agents and can present in many ways. Symptoms may range from a minor inconvenience to severe acute abdominal pain occasionally requiring hospital admission, sometimes surgical intervention. Pelvic infection occurs mainly in sexually active individuals and is uncommon following the menopause. Vaginal discharge in a postmenopausal woman is highly suspicious and should always be investigated fully. Endometrial cancer may present in this way. Risk factors for pelvic infections include multiple sexual partners, the use of an intrauterine contraceptive device (IUCD), and the insertion of foreign bodies into the vagina, including tampons and pessaries.

Although all infections are associated with sexual activity, some are transmitted exclusively by sexual contact. These may also be asymptomatic and screening of high risk individuals such as those attending departments of genito-urinary medicine or seeking termination of pregnancy is extremely important. It is essential in the management of most pelvic infections that the sexual partner is also treated to prevent reinfection. Contact tracing may also be necessary and is best done in a hospital setting.

Presenting symptoms and signs may include:
- offensive vaginal discharge;
- abnormal vaginal bleeding;
- pelvic pain;
- dyspareunia;
- vulval or urethral soreness or the presence of lumps, blisters or warts.

In severe untreated cases generalized symptoms and signs of infection such as rigors and a high temperature may be associated with peritonitis and abscess formation. Vaginal examination may suggest a specific infection from the presence of blisters or warts, or the 'fishy' smell of a discharge due to *Gardnerella* infection. Pelvic examination which reveals cervical excitation and the presence of a tender mass strongly suggests pelvic inflammatory disease (PID).

Investigations should include vaginal, cervical and urethral swabs, where appropriate, for culture and staining and the specific therapy will depend upon the results.

Commonly presenting infections, clinical features and treatments are described in the following sections.

### *Candida*

*Presentation.* 'Vaginal thrush' is a very common infection, experienced by most women at least once in their lives. It is caused by *Candida albicans*. Other species of *Candida* may cause vaginitis, and may be isolated from high vaginal swabs, but are not responsive to standard antifungal treatments. Men may carry penile candidiasis with no symptoms.

Thrush usually presents as vulval or vaginal soreness, accompanied by a thick curdy white discharge. The patient often recognizes it and has had it herself before. Her partner may have an itchy or sore penis.

In recurrent cases, attacks often come on premenstrually, and may be precipitated by sexual intercourse. Very localized itching or soreness, accompanied by an offensive discharge, or recurrent attacks postmenstrually is suggestive of other causes such as *bacterial vaginosis*.

*Candida* may be precipitated by antibiotic treatment particularly broad spectrum antibiotics, the oral contraceptive pill or pregnancy.

*Diagnosis* can often be made from the history alone, particularly if the patient has had it before. Visual inspection may reveal a curdy discharge adherent to the vaginal walls. A sample may be observed directly under the microscope or sent for culture.

The vaginal pH in a healthy individual or a person with *Candida* will usually be lower than five, whereas a pH higher than five is suggestive of bacterial vaginosis or trichomoniasis. Cervical smears are sometimes reported as showing evidence of *Candida*.

*Treatment* is by antifungal agents vaginally such as nystatin, clotrimazole, miconazole or econazole which offer cure rates of 80–90%. Oral treatment such as fluconazole or ketoconazole may be preferred by some women and may be appropriate in severe cases. Oral treatment is not recommended during pregnancy.

In resistant or recurrent cases it is sometimes worthwhile giving prolonged courses of treatment such as clotrimazole 500 mg vaginally on day eight and day 18 of the cycle for several cycles or a combination of oral ketoconazole for five days and miconazole pessaries (100 mg) for 14 days. Depot progesterone may be useful in preventing recurrent thrush, especially if there is a history of thrush having cleared up completely whilst breast-feeding.

### Gardnerella

*Presentation.* Vulval or vaginal soreness, if present at all, is slight compared with *Candida* infection. A watery discharge with a 'fishy' odour may, however, be complained of. The smell is often most pungent after sexual intercourse.

*Diagnosis.* 'Clue cells' may be identified on direct microscopy. The organism may be grown on culture.

*Treatment.* Metronidazole 400 mg twice daily for seven days or 2 g as a single dose to patient and partner.

## Trichomonas vaginalis

*Presentation.* Frothy offensive yellow-green discharge, dysuria, occasionally urethral discharge, occasionally vulval or vaginal soreness.

*Diagnosis.* Direct microscopy, culture of vaginal and/or urethral swabs.

*Treatment.* Metronidazole 400 mg twice daily for seven days of 2 g as a single dose to patient and partner.

## Herpes simplex, type 2

*Presentation.* Genital ulcers often causing extreme pain and tenderness, sometimes making it very uncomfortable for the patient to stand, walk or sit. Occasionally leads to acute retention of urine. Although it may be recurrent, the first episode is often the worst.

*Diagnosis.* Usually made on appearance of genital ulcers and severity of symptoms. Electron microscopy of smears taken from the ulcers will reveal the virus which can also be cultured if transported to the laboratory in viral culture transport medium.

*Treatment.* Oral acyclovir, 200 mg five times daily for five days for adults. Possible hospital admission.

In pregnancy the fetus can be infected during labour and delivery. If an active lesion is present at the time of labour, delivery by caesarean section is recommended within four hours of rupture of the membranes. Infection is unlikely to be transmitted in this way except during a first attack but if in doubt electron microscopy of smears from suspicious lesions at the onset of labour may be helpful.

### Human papilloma virus

*Presentation.* Genital warts, usually painless.

*Diagnosis.* Appearance with or without biopsy.

*Treatment.* Topical podophyllin (podophyllotoxin 0.5%, applied daily for three days, repeating after an interval of four days, for a maximum of five weeks).

Occasionally cryocautery, diathermy, laser vaporization, intralesional interferon or systemic interferon (rarely) may be required.

### Neisseria gonorrhoea

*Presentation.* Gonorrhoea is often asymptomatic and commonly picked up when screening high-risk patients (see above).

Dysuria or urethral discharge may be present in cases of acute urethritis. Soreness of the vulva or vagina, lower abdominal pain and tenderness, suggestive of PID may be present.

*Diagnosis.* Urethral and endocervical swabs for Gram staining, also swabs in charcoal medium for culture.

*Treatment.* Amoxycillin 3 g single dose or Ciprofloxacin 250 mg single dose.

### Chlamydia

*Presentation.* Like gonorrhoea, *Chlamydia* is often asymptomatic, or is detected on investigation of symptoms such as pelvic pain.

*Diagnosis.* Urethral and endocervical swabs in special *Chlamydia* culture transport medium.

*Treatment.* Doxycycline.

## Acute pelvic inflammatory disease

The presence of acute pelvic infection usually gives rise to systemic upset including fever, rigors and a tachycardia. Bilateral lower abdominal pain may be severe and may radiate through to the back. An offensive vaginal discharge may be present and abnormal vaginal bleeding may occur. The patient may be dehydrated.

Abdominal tenderness and guarding, accompanied by cervical excitation and occasionally a pelvic mass make the diagnosis likely. The most important differential diagnosis is an ectopic pregnancy. A sensitive pregnancy test, both urinary and serum may be helpful as well as a transvaginal ultrasound scan. Swabs should be taken and treatment commenced with antibiotics, intravenously if necessary, usually doxycycline and metronidazole. The commonest causative agent is *Chlamydia trachomatous* although *Neisseria gonnorhoeae* often causes a more severe illness. If a pelvic abscess is present it may not require immediate surgical drainage unless it is particularly large or the patient has peritonitis. If after 48 hours there is no shrinkage of an abscess then drainage is usually performed. Occasionally pelvic abscesses may be caused by actinomycosis in association with an IUCD.

## Complications of pelvic infection

### Ectopic pregnancy

A consequence of pelvic infection is damage to the tubal epithelium, in particular cilial damage results in decreased tubal motility, and as most fertilizations occur in the tube there is a high risk of tubal implantation. In addition, the tubes may be distorted by adhesions forming in the pelvis making transport of the fertilized ovum more difficult.

## Infertility

For the same reasons as those given for ectopic pregnancy, failure to conceive may be a late complication of PID. Tubal transport may be compromised and the lumen may even be occluded following infection, making it difficult even at operation to make the tubes patent again. Adhesions may also prevent release of the ovum into the tube.

## Cervical neoplasia

The presence of wart virus infection is associated with both preinvasive and invasive malignancy of the cervix. There is no treatment available to eradicate the wart virus and it is therefore most important that regular cervical smears are taken. Currently it is only recommended that smears are done every three years unless the presence of the wart virus has been seen to be associated with dyskaryosis.

## Pelvic pain

Perhaps the most distressing long-term complication of PID is chronic pelvic pain associated with intermittent acute infective flare-ups. The pain can be extremely debilitating and analgesics are often ineffective. The only certain cure is pelvic clearance with hysterectomy and bilateral salpingo-oöphorectomy, otherwise the difficult problem of a 'frozen pelvis' arises. When pelvic clearance is undertaken in young women long-term hormone replacement therapy (HRT) should be considered.

## Toxic shock syndrome

This is due to a toxin produced by *Staphylococcus aureus*, which in gynaecological practice is usually associated with a retained tampon. A retained tampon may present to the general practitioner as a discharge or abnormal bleeding, or the patient may think that she has lost a tampon. When removed there is a highly pungent malodorous lingering smell. If a tampon is retained unknowingly, the patient may present with a high fever, dizziness, vomiting, hypotension and possibly a rash due to thrombocytopaenia. Renal, cardiac and pulmonary complications may follow. Investigations may reveal abnormalities of the white cell and platelet count as well as renal and hepatic disturbances. Treatment is usually removal of the retained tampon, rehydration and intravenous flucloxacillin.

## Questions

**Q1**: How common is genital herpes and how should it be managed and by whom? Is genital herpes during pregnancy a cause for concern?

**A**: A general practitioner with a list size of 2000 patients will expect to see about two new cases of genital herpes each year. Its presentation can be genuinely described as an emergency because it is so extremely painful. If the patient presents in surgery she may have difficulty in walking and difficulty in urinating. The primary attack is often said to be the worst and most painful. Primary or secondary attacks respond well to acyclovir or famciclovir, but oral analgesia may be required also. Topical treatments are probably ineffective. Consideration should be given to: referral to a genito-urinary medicine department for follow-up; screening for other associated infections and advice regarding cervical smear follow-up, usually recommended annually.

Active genital herpes at the time of delivery is considered a reason for delivery by caesarean section to avoid infection reaching the neonate. A primary attack of genital herpes during pregnancy can affect the fetus and close consultation with the consultant obstetrician is essential.

**Q2**: In the management of women with recurrent thrush, should the male partner also receive treatment?

**A1**: If the male partner has candidal balanitis it would obviously be worthwhile offering him treatment. Therefore if the problem is recurrent thrush it would probably be worthwhile seeing the male partner and offering treatment. Men can carry *Candida* and remain asymptomatic and although there would, in these circumstances, be no harm in treating, co-treatment of the male partner does not appear to reduce the relapse rate.

# 9: Common Gynaecological Malignancies

Malignant disease can arise in the vulva, vagina, cervix uterine body, fallopian tubes or ovaries. Carcinoma affecting the vagina or fallopian tubes is extremely rare and it is uncommon in the vulva. Similar numbers of new cases of cancer of the ovary, endometrium and uterine cervix occur in the UK each year, but deaths due to ovarian cancer are double those due to the other two.

## Cervical cancer

The majority of cervical cancers are squamous lesions arising in the transformation zone (see Chapter 10, Cervical Screening and Colposcopy). Although there are an increasing number of adenocarcinomas and mixed tumours.

### Predisposing factors

These include smoking, wart virus infection, multiple sexual partners and an early age of first sexual intercourse. The cervical screening programme is widely established but has only recently appeared to be making an impact upon the incidence of invasive disease, largely because people at the highest risk of cervical cancer have been least good at being screened for the disease.

Cervical cancer occurs in all age groups, although it is very rare under the age of 20 years. There are two age peaks of incidence, in the late 30s and 50s.

### Presentation

The main early symptoms of cervical cancer are abnormal

vaginal bleeding and/or vaginal discharge. *Cervical precancers are generally asymptomatic* and are diagnosed on cervical cytology and/or colposcopy (see Chapter 10).

Invasive disease of the cervix cannot be diagnosed with certainty on cervical cytology alone as this involves only the removal of the surface epithelium in taking a cervical smear whereas invasion of the cervix is dependant upon the breaching of the basement membrane to establish the diagnosis. There are however certain cytological features which may be suggestive of invasive disease.

In the premenopausal woman symptoms of invasive carcinoma may present with abnormal vaginal bleeding following intercourse, or it may occur intermenstrually with complete cycle regularity. A bloodstained discharge may also be present.

Clinical examination of the cervix with a speculum may show a friable or ulcerated lesion which bleeds easily on contact. The cervix may be mobile or fixed, depending upon the stage of the disease. Cervical cytology is often unhelpful in these circumstances and smears may often be reported as inflammatory or technically unsuitable.

*Concern about the appearance of the cervix should prompt a much more urgent referral than the presence of severe dyskaryosis in a macroscopically normal looking cervix.*

Pain is often a late symptom in cervical cancer and is usually only present in advanced disease.

### Management of cervical cancer

If there is any doubt whatsoever about the diagnosis, the patient should undergo colposcopy. If there is a suspicion of invasive cancer on colposcopy, a cone biopsy should be undertaken. *If invasive cancer is obviously present then the disease should be staged.*

The staging of cervical cancer is clinical and is based upon findings after examination under anaesthetic, involving cystoscopy, cervical biopsy and rectal examination to assess lateral spread. Proctoscopy and intravenous pyelography are also allowed. Endometrial curettage should be undertaken; whilst spread to the body of uterus does not alter the staging there is some suggestion that with spread to the body of the uterus the prognosis is less good.

The International Federation of Gynaecology and Obstetrics (FIGO) classification of staging is as follows.

Stage 1A (part 1)   Micro-invasive disease only just breaking through the basement membrane.

Stage 1A (part 2)   Micro-invasive disease, maximum depth of invasion of 5 mm with a maximum surface diameter of 7 mm, not clinically suspicious.

Stage 1B (occult)   More advanced than 1A part 2, and not clinically obvious.

Stage 1B   Disease confined to the cervix.

Stage 2A and B   Spread to the upper two-thirds of the vagina (2A) or parametrium but not reaching the pelvic sidewall (2B).

Stage 3A and B   Spread to the lower third of the vagina (3A), pelvic sidewall (3B) or hydronephrosis (3C).

Stage 4A and B   Spread to the mucosa of the bladder or the rectum (4A), or spread beyond the pelvis (4B).

### Treatment

Treatment depends upon the stage of the disease. Stage 1A part 1 and 1A part 2 to a depth of 3 mm can be safely managed by complete local excision, usually cone biopsy, assuming that there is no lymphatic involvement or vascular channel involvement. Stage 1 disease beyond this and stage 2A (spread to the upper two-thirds of the vagina only) may be managed either by radical surgery or radiotherapy.

Stages 2B to 4A are usually managed by pelvic irradiation, whilst the management of stage 4B disease is palliative only.

The results of surgery and radiotherapy in stages 1B and 2A are similar and the choice of treatment is dictated by the patient's age as well as the size and grade of tumour. The advantages of extended hysterectomy and pelvic lymphadenectomy over radiotherapy are that the ovaries can be spared in the former and there is less interference with vaginal function. A surgical approach is therefore usually favoured in pre-menopausal women. If the lymph nodes are involved with the tumour following surgical removal, then pelvic radiotherapy is usually undertaken as part of the treatment.

In stages 1B and 2A, if there are risk factors for lymph node involvement such as a large tumour or one that is poorly differentiated, then radiotherapy may be preferred to surgery.

The treatment of recurrent disease depends upon the site of the recurrence, as well as previous treatment, but may involve radiotherapy, exenterative surgery (rarely) or chemotherapy. Chemotherapy seems to have a very limited role in cervical cancer.

## *Prognosis*

The prognosis for cervical cancer depends upon the stage at initial presentation (see above). The approximate five-year survival rates are as follows.

| | |
|---|---|
| Stage 1 (with negative lymph nodes) | 80% |
| Stage 1 (with positive lymph nodes) | 60% |
| Stage 2 | 50% |
| Stage 3 | 30% |
| Stage 4 | 10% |

## Endometrial cancer

Most cancers arising in the endometrium are adenocarcinomas. The majority occur in postmenopausal women although there is an increasing incidence in women around the age of 40 years. It is rare under the age of 40 years.

*Any woman over the age of 40 years presenting with irregular cycles and intermenstrual bleeding should be referred for dilatation and curettage (D&C).* Whilst the majority of women presenting in this way will have dysfunctional uterine bleeding (DUB) a small minority will have endometrial cancer.

### Predisposing factors

These include obesity, nulliparity, diabetes and the use of un-opposed oestrogens.

### Presentation

In postmenopausal women the disease presents with vaginal bleeding or discharge. Vaginal infection causing bleeding is much less common after the menopause than in younger women and anyone with postmenopausal bleeding or discharge should be referred.

Before the menopause, women present with irregular periods and intermenstrual bleeding.

Cervical cytology may occasionally detect adenocarcinomatous cells but their absence does not exclude the diagnosis of endometrial cancer.

Clinical examination is often unhelpful except when bleeding is clearly visualized from the cervical os.

The commonest cause of postmenopausal bleeding is *atrophic vaginitis* but this diagnosis may only be safely made when other more serious pathology has been excluded.

### Management

If there is sufficient clinical suspicion of endometrial malignancy, diagnostic curettage must be performed. Hysteroscopy allows direct visualization of the endometrial cavity which may reveal a small lesion which could easily be missed during a 'blind' curettage. Hysteroscopy can also be helpful in staging the disease.

The FIGO classification of endometrial cancer is as follows.

Stage 1     Confined to the uterine corpus.
Stage 1A    Limited to the endometrium.
Stage 1B    Invasion of less than half of the myometrium.
Stage 1C    Invasion of more than half of the myometrium.
Stage 2     Involving the uterine cervix.
Stage 2A    Endocervical glandular involvement only.
Stage 2B    Cervical stromal invasion.
Stage 3A    Tumour involves serosa and/or adnexae and/or positive peritoneal cytology.
Stage 3B    Metastases to pelvic and/or para-aortic lymph nodes.
Stage 4A    Tumour invasion of bladder or bowel mucosa.
Stage 4B    Distant metastases including intra-abdominal and/or inguinal lymph nodes.

Although patients with endometrial cancer may be poor operative risks, the mainstay of treatment nevertheless is surgical.

In stages 1 and 2 disease, a total abdominal hysterectomy and bilateral salpingo-oöphorectomy is usually performed with postoperative pelvic radiotherapy being reserved for those at high risk of lymphatic involvement, e.g. those with high-grade tumours and those invading deeply into the myometrium.

In stage 3 disease the treatment of choice is surgical resection of all the disease as far as is possible combined with postoperative pelvic radiotherapy with or without progesterone therapy.

The management of stage 4 disease depends on the site and the amount of disease but it is often palliative with hormonal therapy.

Cytotoxic treatment has a very limited place in the treatment of endometrial cancer. In patients who are a very poor operative risk, radiotherapy may be used as primary treatment though the results are less good than with surgery.

## Prognosis

The approximate five-year survival rates for endometrial cancer are as follows.

Stage 1      80%
Stage 2      50%
Stage 3      30%
Stage 4      10%

## Ovarian cancer

Ovarian cancer is the fifth most common malignancy in women and is the most common gynaecological malignancy in the UK. There are approximately twice as many deaths per year due to ovarian cancer than deaths due to cervical cancer. Unfortunately no ideal screening test exists for ovarian cancer, though serum tumour markers such as CA125 and ovariectomized (OVX) 1, together with transvaginal ultrasound and pelvic examination, are currently undergoing nationwide trials.

The prognosis for ovarian cancer is poor with the overall five-year survival rate of less than 25%. This survival rate is much increased when the disease is localized within the ovary but most cases present clinically with symptoms when spread has already often occurred into the peritoneum.

The majority of ovarian malignancies are epithelial tumours. Occasionally other types of tumour arise such as germ cell tumours, functioning tumours and others including secondary deposits.

Epithelial tumours of the ovary are rare under the age of 40 years, but germ cell tumours often arise in younger women. Any young woman presenting with an ovarian cyst may have a germ cell tumour and serum tumour markers should be measured preoperatively in case this turns out to be the case, because tumour markers are extremely useful in monitoring follow-up.

### Risk factors for ovarian cancer

*Increased risk*
1 Increasing age, especially over the age of 45 years.
2 Nulliparity.
3 Investigation and treatment for infertility.
4 A personal history of breast, endometrial or colonic cancer.
5 A family history of ovarian cancer in a first degree relative. A positive family history of ovarian cancer in one first degree relative increases the individual patient's risk to 5%. If two first degree relatives are affected, the individual patient's risk is increased to 30%.

*The overall risk of breast cancer in women with NO positive family history is 10%.*

Jewish and white women have an increased risk of ovarian cancer in comparison to black women in whom it is extremely rare.

*Decreased risk*
1 Any full term pregnancy.
2 The oral contraceptive pill.
3 Breast-feeding.
4 Hysterectomy.
5 Sterilization.

### Presentation

Carcinoma of the ovary results in twice as many deaths per year as cervical and endometrial cancer combined. More than 50% of cases are at stage 3 (see below) at the time of presentation.

Presenting symptoms may be vague such as anorexia, dyspepsia and altered bowel habit and extensive investigation of the gastro-intestinal tract is not uncommon before the diagnosis of ovarian cancer is reached. Often ovarian tumours are picked up because of abdominal swelling and bloating at an advanced stage.

Abnormal vaginal bleeding may be a presenting sign in up to a fifth of cases and the diagnosis of ovarian cancer should always be considered if other investigations such as D&C prove negative.

Because of the often late presentation of ovarian cancer, screening for the disease has been and is being researched (see above) but so far the available screening tools are neither sensitive or specific enough to be widely used. In addition the natural history of the development of ovarian cancer is not fully understood and so the relevance of tumour markers (CA125 and OVX 1) are still not clear. Tumour markers can, however, be extremely useful in the follow-up of patients after treatment.

Furthermore, the follow-up of patients with positive or suspiciously high tests is to undergo surgery, laparoscopy or laparotomy, both of which carry some risk themselves.

Perhaps screening women with one or more first degree relatives with a history of the disease is worthwhile and these women may even wish to consider bilateral oöphorectomy once their family is completed.

## Management

The treatment of ovarian cancer is by laparotomy with hysterectomy, bilateral salpingo-oöphorectomy, infracolic omentectomy (the commonest extrapelvic site of spread) and by the debulking of any other tumour with the aim of leaving behind as little disease as possible. As well as removing as much disease as possible, the laparotomy also serves to clinically stage and plan adjuvant therapy, which is most likely to be successful with minimal residual tumour.

Unfortunately, the long-term results of such treatment are poor (the overall five-year survival rate is less than 25%) and as a consequence the role of initial surgery has been called into question with the suggestion that as soon as a tissue diagnosis has been made, aggressive chemotherapy may be just as effective. This however, still remains to be established and the current suggested best management remains surgical removal and debulking of as much tumour as possible, followed by chemotherapy in all except those unfit to undergo such treatment, and those with stage 1A or 1B disease (see below).

The staging of ovarian cancer is as follows.

Stage 1A    Limited to one ovary, no ascites, no tumour on the external surface of the ovary, capsule intact.

Stage 1B    As above but involving both ovaries.

Stage 1C    As above but the tumour extending to external surface, capsule ruptured, or positive washings or ascites.

Stage 2     Involving one or both ovaries with pelvic extension.

Stage 3     Tumour spreading beyond pelvis in the peritoneal cavity plus or minus retroperitoneal or inguinal nodes plus or minus superficial liver secondaries.

Stage 4     Distant metastases or parenchymal liver disease.

Following initial surgery, adjuvant treatment would be indicated in stages 2 to 4. Most oncologists would not however give further treatment in stages 1A and B and some would not give further treatment in stage 1C.

In the UK the main form of adjuvant therapy is either single-agent platinum-based therapy or combination chemotherapy including platinum.

Radiotherapy is not widely favoured in this country as it has to be given to the whole abdomen and is often associated with significant morbidity. The best chance of cure or worthwhile remission from ovarian cancer is aggressive initial treatment.

With recurrent disease, further chemotherapy, surgery or radiotherapy may be offered but the results are generally unsatisfactory. It is important with any malignancy, especially ovarian cancer, to be able to judge when to withdraw aggressive treatment and commence palliative care.

## Palliative care

The treatment of the dying patient is extremely demanding and involves caring for both the physical and psychological needs of the patient and her family. Most often a multi-disciplinary approach involving the gynaecologist, oncologist, radiotherapist and specialist in palliative care will provide the optimum care. Pain relief, management of nausea and vomiting, bowel problems, tissue necrosis, haemorrhage and infection are all common problems requiring careful medical and nursing skills. The options of care at home, in hospital or in a hospice should all be considered, assisting the patient to make an informed choice.

## Prognosis

The approximate five-year survival rate in *epithelial* ovarian cancer is as follows.

Stage 1     70%
Stage 2     50%
Stage 3     30%
Stage 4     <10%

The above reference has been made to epithelial tumours. In addition the following types of tumours may occur.

## Borderline tumours

Epithelial tumours may be benign or malignant, but they can also sometimes be described as borderline. Borderline tumours have all the features of malignancy, except that there is no stromal invasion. The diagnosis cannot be made until after surgery and the initial treatment is the same as for invasive disease. There is no conclusive evidence to suggest that chemotherapy or radiotherapy have any role in the initial treatment of these lesions even if they are at an advanced stage. They can recur following surgery and patients will require careful follow-up.

## Other ovarian tumours

### Functioning ovarian tumours

These secrete androgens or oestrogens and may present with hormonal manifestations such as *hirsutism*. They are managed surgically.

### Germ cell tumours

These are extremely sensitive to chemotherapy with excellent cure rates. In stage 1A disease unilateral oöphorectomy followed by careful monitoring of tumour markers (CA125 and OVX1) or chemotherapy will usually result in cure. In more advanced disease surgical debulking followed by chemotherapy is the treatment of choice.

## The United Kingdom Cancer Family Study

The CRC Human Cancer Genetic Research Group at Cambridge is running an ongoing United Kingdom Cancer Family Study group and a UK CCCR Familial Ovarian Cancer Study. Any family with two or more first or second degree relatives who have had epithelial ovarian cancer are eligible for the trial which will consist of pelvic examination, transvaginal ultrasound and serum markers. If results are negative the screening will be offered in one year's time; if positive a second more sensitive ultrasound examination will be offered before surgical exploration. The age range for eligible women is between 25 (or five years below the age of the youngest case in the family if this is younger) and 70 years.

## Questions

**Q1**: Who should be screened for ovarian cancer?

**A**: As yet no ideal screening tool exists, furthermore there is no preinvasive (treatable, perhaps curable) stage and there is as yet no evidence that screening reduces mortality.

**Q2**: How reliable are tumour markers in the diagnosis and follow-up of women with ovarian cancer?

**A**: No single reliable serum tumour marker exists. The most commonly used at present are:

• carcinoembryonic antigen (CEA), 50% of women with ovarian cancer have raised levels, 50% do not; following treatment for ovarian cancer (see above) a rising titre indicates recurrence is likely;

• CA125 is raised in most cases of ovarian cancer (high sensitivity) but is also raised in other cancers and in endometriosis (low specificity).

**Q3**: What are the commonest side-effects of pelvic irradiation?

**A**: The main problems are short-term bladder and bowel morbidity. These are usually self-limiting but can become chronic problems. Occasionally serious complications such as fistulae may develop.

# 10: Cervical Screening and Colposcopy

The annual incidence of invasive cervical cancer in the UK has been approximately 4000 cases over recent years with approximately 2000 deaths per annum. There has been and continues to be debate on the effectiveness of screening for cervical cancer in this country due to the failure of screening to appear to have any effect upon incidence of the disease. The most likely explanation for this is failure to screen the high risk population. With the introduction of nationwide computerized call and recall systems, the incidence of new cases appears to be declining.

For any meaningful and successful screening programme, several criteria should be observed (Koch's postulates).

**1** The condition must be relatively common causing significant morbidity or mortality within the population being screened.

**2** The natural history of the condition must be fully understood in order to establish desired frequency of screening and to establish that early intervention will result in a significant improvement in outcome.

**3** The screening test must be effective, acceptable and generally applicable to the population being screened.

**4** The test should be sensitive (i.e. few false negative test results) and specific (i.e. few false positive results).

**5** The screening programme should be cost-effective.

The Papanicolaou smear test meets these criteria and is used to detect precancer cells.

It is widely believed that most cases of invasive cervical cancer arise in pre-existing preinvasive cancers known as cervical intraepithelial neoplasia (CIN).

There are three grades of CIN, and it is believed that about 50% of CIN III lesions will progress to invasion if left untreated. The usual progression rate from onset of CIN to invasion is probably about 10 years but there appear to be certain cases of a much more aggressive lesion.

The smear test is taken by inserting a speculum, usually a bivalve Cusco's speculum, into the vagina in order to visualize the cervix. A wooden spatula is inserted into the cervical canal and rotated through 360° in order to sample cells from the ectocervix (that part of the cervix which is visible) and the endocervical canal. The sample is then smeared onto a named glass slide and immediately 'fixed' in alcohol before sending to the laboratory.

At the laboratory the slide is treated with a Papanicolaou stain prior to microscopic examination, which takes about 15 minutes.

The aim of taking a smear is to sample squamous cells from the ectocervix and columnar cells from the endocervical canal. Absence of either type of cell indicates an unsatisfactory smear, indicating failure to sample the transformation zone. The point at which the squamous and columnar cells meet is called the squamo–columnar junction (SCJ). In young women this tends to be some distance from the external cervical os on the ectocervix and it gradually moves towards and then into the canal by a process of squamous metaplasia as well as cervical inversion.

Squamous metaplasia, the process by which columnar cells change into squamous cells, occurs most actively around the time of birth, at the menarche and during the first pregnancy. Certain trigger factors, including smoking and the presence of the wart virus infection, can cause the metabolic process to become dysplastic with the formation of premalignant and ultimately malignant lesions. The SCJ tends to disappear into the cervical canal around the time of the menopause. The area between the original and the current SCJ is the transformation zone and this is the region in which the majority of squamous lesions (CIN) occur.

Glandular abnormalities which may ultimately become

adenocarcinomas arise from columnar epithelium above the SCJ.

Endocervical cells give rise to an ectropion.

## Problems with smears

Problems with the smear test may arise from inadequate sampling or incorrect interpretation, and some studies have reported false negative results as high as 20%. Because of this it is recommended that the second smear is performed one year after the first ever smear, and then at three-yearly intervals until the age of 65 years.

The current recommendations are that screening should be carried out selectively in teenagers who are at high risk, for example those who are attending genito-urinary clinics, those who began to have sexual intercourse at an early age and women with many sexual partners. Whole population screening should begin in all sexually active women from the age of 20 years.

Three-yearly screening, after the initial two smears separated by one year, has been shown to be cost-effective, with the additional pick-up rate not able to justify the extra cost of more frequent screening (see Table 10.1).

## Smear reports

The following reports, or similar, may be issued by the laboratory, and the appropriate action is necessary.

**Table 10.1** The 'pick-up' rate for detection of abnormalities at cervical screening, by periodicity.

| Screening frequency (years) | Prevention of cervical carcinoma (%) |
|---|---|
| 5 | 84 |
| 3 | 91 |
| 1 | 93 |

*Negative, satisfactory smear.* Continue screening at routine intervals, i.e. three-yearly after two initial negative smears separated by one year.

*Inadequate smear or technically unsuitable.* Repeat test in three months. If still unsuitable refer for colposcopy.

*Inflammatory smear.* It may be worthwhile asking the local laboratory what is meant by this. In the absence of specific guidelines, take high vaginal and endocervical swabs, in Stuarts' medium and *Chlamydia* culture medium, and treat any infection appropriately, then repeat the cervical smear in three months time. If the woman is postmenopausal, she may require oestrogen, either topically or orally (as well as proges- terone if she still has a uterus) before repeating the smear in three to six months time. If the smear remains inflammatory after three months refer for colposcopy.

*Borderline nuclear abnormality or wart virus infection.* If re- ported the cervical smear should be repeated in six months. If the same abnormality persists, refer for colposcopy.

*Mild dyskaryosis.* Until recently the recommendation has been to repeat the test in six months. *Recent data suggests that all mild dyskaryosis should be referred immediately for colpo- scopy,* although there is still considerable debate about this.

*Moderate/severe dyskaryosis.* Refer for colposcopy.

*Atypical glandular cells.* Refer for colposcopy.

*Invasive carcinoma.* Refer for urgent colposcopy.

*Koilocytes.* Cells with a halo around the nucleus indicative of infection with human papilloma virus (HPV). Repeat in six months and *refer for colposcopy if still present.*

*Actinomyces or actinomyces-like organisms* (ALOs). These are sometimes seen in women with IUCDs. Most often women are asymptomatic but the coil should be removed, an alternative method of contraception employed, and the smear repeated in three months time. A coil can be re-inserted if this smear is normal.

Because of the natural history of cervical cancer, a pre-malignant change is unlikely to develop into an invasive lesion in a short period of time. Usually, if the cervix looks macroscopically normal at the time of the smear being taken, the need for colposcopic assessment is not urgent unless a report of invasive carcinoma is received. However, because of the anxiety caused to the patient, the waiting time for colposcopic examination should be kept to a minimum.

A cervical smear which is suggestive of invasive carcinoma is not certain until confirmed by biopsies. A cervical smear samples only those cells on the surface of the epithelium, and a firm diagnosis of invasive carcinoma is dependent upon histology confirming penetration of the basement membrane.

Concern about the appearance of the cervix, particularly if associated with symptoms such as postcoital or intermenstrual bleeding, and even without a smear suggesting dyskaryosis is in much more urgent need of colposcopic assessment than a routine cervical smear from a macroscopically normal cervix showing severe dyskaryosis. Dyskaryotic cells from an invasive carcinoma may be masked on a smear by a lot of inflammatory cells and such smears should be repeated, after treatment if appropriate or advised (see above).

*Dyskaryosis* refers to abnormalities of individual cells, whilst *dysplasia* is a tissue diagnosis, such as CIN III. The correlation between smear abnormalities and tissue diagnosis is generally poor.

## Correlation between cytology and colposcopic histology

Mild dyskaryosis      CIN I
Moderate dyskaryosis   CIN II
Severe dyskaryosis     CIN III

In clinical practice, the actual correlation has been found to be less accurate.

## Colposcopy

Colposcopy is a more detailed assessment of the cervix using binocular magnification of about 7–10 times. A speculum is passed to allow visualization of the cervix and upper vagina. After naked eye inspection looking for areas of leukoplakia or abnormal blood vessels, a solution of 5% acetic acid is applied to the cervix. This causes precipitation of cytoplasmic protein in abnormal cells resulting in a white appearance of varying grades. The white areas may be interspersed with areas of mosaicism or punctuation indicating abnormal vessel formation and usually a higher-grade lesion. It is important to assess the degree of abnormality as well as its extent particularly if the SCJ can be fully visualized (columnar epithelium has the appearance of 'bunches of grapes' through the colposcope). The following management procedures should be followed.

### Whole lesion seen, no suspicion of invasion

1 Punch biopsy to confirm CIN and then destructive treatment with laser, cold coagulation or diathermy; or
2 punch biopsy to confirm CIN followed by excisional treatment with loop diathermy or laser; or
3 initial excisional treatment as above at first visit if sure that treatment is necessary.

In general, excisional treatment is favoured because of reports of late recurrences of invasive carcinomas after initial destructive treatments when excision may have indicated an early occult invasive lesion.

*Whole lesion not seen (squamo–columnar junction not visible)*

Cone biopsy should be performed in view of the risk of an invasive lesion present in the endocervical canal. The cone biopsy may be performed with a scalpel or with loop diathermy.

*Suspicion of invasive carcinoma*

A cone biopsy should be performed to excise the whole lesion widely. This procedure may be performed with a scalpel or loop diathermy, usually under general anaesthesia to ensure that a satisfactory specimen is obtained.

*Obvious (macroscopic appearance) invasive carcinoma*

Wedge biopsy and staging should be undertaken (see Chapter 9 on Common Gynaecological Malignancies).

*Atypical glandular cells seen on cervical smear*

The cervical smear should be repeated at the time of colposcopy. If atypical glandular cells are still present, then cone biopsy with endometrial sampling should be performed as the lesion must be arising above the SCJ within the endocervical canal. There may be a coexisting lesion on the ectocervix.

At the time of colposcopy the upper vagina must also be assessed because failure to identify and treat vaginal extension of CIN initially is likely to cause significant management difficulties later.

Following colposcopy and appropriate treatment, follow-up should be with cervical cytology at six months and then annually for five years. Thereafter, if there is no sign of recurrence, routine follow-up at three-yearly intervals should take place. If resources permit, the first two assessments following treatment should include further colposcopy.

Following excisional treatment, the histology report on the specimen may show CIN extending to one margin. It is not necessary following this report to proceed to further treatment because in more than 50% of cases there will be no residual disease, and any previously abnormal cells may be destroyed in the inflammatory response around the excision crater on the cervix. If there is residual or early recurrent disease, further treatment either with cone biopsy or hysterectomy may be necessary. *Following hysterectomy, if the vaginal margins are free from abnormal cells, follow-up vault smears should be at six months and 18 months after hysterectomy.* If these are both normal no further screening is necessary.

Residual or recurrent disease at the vaginal vault is more difficult to treat but further surgery or radiotherapy may be appropriate.

Abnormalities occurring on the cervix some time after the original treatment require careful colposcopic assessment and are usually best managed by cone biopsy using a scalpel as the extent of the lesion is more difficult to assess following previous therapy.

## Questions

**Q1**: How frequently should a woman with genital warts have a cervical smear?

**A**: Genital warts (condylomata acuminata) are usually painless pink or grey swellings which are usually pedunculated or sessile and can appear anywhere on the external genitalia, perineum, urethra or cervix. Ano-genital warts are caused by human papilloma virus (HPV) types 6, 11, 16 and 18. Types 16 and 18 are associated with carcinoma of the cervix. If repeat cervical smears show persistant HPV infection, the patient should be referred for colposcopy. If colposcopy does not reveal associated CIN, then the patient can be returned to the normal screening programme, otherwise appropriate treatment will be required.

Advice from the local laboratory and gynaecological services should be sought in difficult cases.

Twenty per cent of patients with a genital wart have another sexually transmitted disease (STD).

**Q2**: Should a bimanual examination always be undertaken at the time of a routine cervical smear?

**A**: In theory the answer is 'yes' but in practice it is rare to pick up any unsuspected pelvic pathology in an asymptomatic woman presenting for a cervical smear.

**Q3**: What are the advantages of loop diathermy of the cervix versus laser ablation following abnormalities discovered at colposcopy?

**A**: The loop diathermy method provides a histological specimen to confirm that no occult invasive lesion is present. Patients undergoing loop diathermy can be sent back to the general practitioner more quickly for follow-up, usually by cervical smear, whereas patients treated with laser tend to require longer follow-up at hospital out-patient departments and will require further colposcopy.

# 11: New Developments in Gynaecology

There are a number of important areas of change in gynaecological practice that are currently evolving. Some of these changes, such as an increasing number of day-case surgical procedures have direct implications on selection of suitable patients for referral and follow-up care in the community. As in other surgical specialties, the precise role of minimal access surgery is yet to be fully defined.

As well as surgery, advances are continuing to be made in both endocrinology and oncology, with an increasing expectation of more prescribing of less familiar drugs.

In addition many new drugs and drug delivery systems have been developed for gynaecological symptoms particularly in the areas of contraception and hormone replacement therapy (HRT).

## Day-case surgery and minimal access surgery

Many gynaecological procedures are now performed as day-cases or at least very short-stay cases. This is advantageous for the patient, providing there are no complications, and also has significant cost-saving advantages to hospital trusts.

Although initially it was felt that the majority of gynaecological procedures would eventually be performed laparoscopically or by hysteroscopy, some of the early enthusiasm has been tempered by unforeseen complications and drawbacks. The following procedures are commonly performed as day-cases and their potential problems are outlined below.

### Dilatation and curettage (D&C)

This is most commonly performed for diagnostic purposes, in

95

premenopausal women with irregular bleeding or in postmenopausal women with bleeding. Normally, women may bleed for a day or two afterwards but should not normally expect to feel pain. Pain or continued bleeding, particularly if heavy, after more than a few days is an indication for a further hospital opinion, as is a raised temperature or offensive vaginal discharge.

## *Hysteroscopy and endometrial ablation*

Hysteroscopy allows a view of the uterine cavity rather than obtaining curettings 'blind'. Pathologies such as polyps, fibroids, adhesions or carcinomas may be visualized. In addition, newer equipment allows inspection of the fallopian tubes which may reveal intrinsic tubal damage which was previously undetectable and therefore untreatable. Ablation of the endometrium, by diathermy laser or cryotherapy, may allow women in their mid to late 40s to avoid hysterectomy.

## *Endometrial resection*

Endometrial resection uses a cutting diathermy loop to resect the endometrium a piece at a time which is quicker than laser ablation and also allows material to be sent for histology. Endometrial resection also carries a slightly greater risk of uterine perforation, although this is likely to be evident before the patient is discharged home from hospital.

After discharge from hospital the patient may take several days to stop bleeding. Thereafter complete amenorrhoea may follow, or the amount of blood loss with each period should at least be reduced to more acceptable levels.

Complications such as those following D&C (listed above) may follow.

### Laparoscopic surgery

Diagnostic laparoscopy and laparoscopic surgery, has been extended from sterilization procedures to drainage of cysts, diathermy of endometrial deposits, division of adhesions, salpingectomy, oöphorectomy, myomectomy and hysterectomy.

It would appear that the management of most ectopic pregnancies can be performed satisfactorily by laparoscopy, some without resort to removal of the tube. Ovarian cystectomies can certainly be performed by laparoscopy and occasionally there are advantages in removing the ovaries laparoscopically at the same time as performing a vaginal hysterectomy.

The role and indications for laparoscopic hysterectomy remains to be defined. One of the big advantages of these new techniques has been a recognition by gynaecologists of the advantage of performing vaginal rather than abdominal hysterectomy wherever possible.

Laparoscopy is a common investigation particularly in cases of infertility and the investigation of pelvic pain.

During the procedure, carbon dioxide is introduced into the abdominal cavity via a subumbilical incision, creating a pneumoperitoneum which allows the safe introduction of a laparoscope into the abdomen via a trochar and cannula.

Postoperatively, apart from minimal discomfort at the incision sites, a bloated abdomen, with discomfort beneath both diaphragms and occasionally referred shoulder tip pain, may be experienced but has usually subsided within 24 hours. If a dye has been used during laparoscopy, for the investigation of tubal patency, this dye may be lost vaginally for a few days afterwards.

### Laser or loop diathermy to the cervix

Most case of cervical intraepithelial neoplasia (CIN) are suitable for local laser ablation or loop diathermy excision, as a day case, using local or general anaesthetic. The patient is often allowed home on the same day and is prescribed topical anti-biotic cream.

The biggest problem postoperatively is bleeding. If this is heavy, particularly in the first few days postoperatively, or 7–10 days postoperatively, the patient may need re-admitting to hospital. There may be a blood-stained vaginal discharge for up to three weeks and the patient should be advised not to use internal tampons and to avoid penetrative sexual intercourse for the first four weeks following the procedure to allow the ectocervix to heal. The period following the procedure should occur around the normal expected time.

### Developments in endocrinology

Most new developments, in this sub-specialty, are in more sophisticated techniques for treating infertility and new developments in preventing conception.

In fertility practice, more specialized forms of *in vitro* fertilization (IVF) are developing, particularly in cases of male infertility. Particular new techniques include subzonal implantation of spermatozoa into the oöcyte, and also computerized selection of sperms for such procedures.

In contraception, the two most interesting developments are the hormonal implants (Norplant, see below) which offers contraception for up to five years, and the addition of progestogens to intrauterine contraceptive devices (IUCDs). The latter method will have a much wider audience than for the existing IUCD, particularly because of its high effective rate and low incidence of side-effects, particularly pelvic infection.

### Developments in oncology

The role of the radical oncological surgeon is declining. The cervical screening programme is at last beginning to have an impact upon the number of new cases of cervical cancer.

In ovarian cancer, the role of prolonged and extensive surgery is being increasingly questioned and the way forward in this disease is more sophisticated chemotherapy, possibly immunotherapy. Unfortunately research into screening for ovarian cancer has yet to provide a satisfactory screening tool which is acceptably sensitive and specific.

The newest and most interesting drugs are Taxol and Taxitere, derived from the yew tree. They both appear to offer advantages in both the initial adjuvant chemotherapy and also in chemotherapy for recurrent disease.

## New products

### Menopausal symptoms

Many new products are emerging for the treatment of menopausal symptoms. The latest developments in this field are included in this section.

The concept of continuous combined therapy (CCT) is not a new one and offers the advantage of achieving amenorrhoea in 80% of women in the first 12 months after an initial phase of irregular bleeding in the first few months. Protection from osteoporosis is optimal, progestogenic side-effects are minimal. Because the pill is a single combination pill of the two hormones, only one prescription charge is payable, whereas in other preparations, consisting of two separate pills, for use at different times in the cycle, two charges are made, one for each item. The only product available at present, Kliofem, is a combination of oestradiol 2 mg and norethisterone 1 mg. It is recommended for the relief of menopausal symptoms in women over the age of 54 years or more than one year since their last menstrual period.

Long-cycle combined HRT has been formulated to relieve the problems of progestogenic side-effects and produce a withdrawal bleed only once each three months. Tridestra combines oestradiol 2 mg for 70 days followed by medroxyprogesterone 20 mg for 14 days followed by 7 placebo days.

New topical HRT preparations include a topical oestradiol gel, Oestrogel, delivered from a pressurized dispenser, usually to the shoulder or thigh areas, providing 24 hours relief from menopausal symptoms.

## Tridestra

Tridestra (Sanofi Winthrop) is a new sequential combined HRT providing a quarterly bleed at the end of each three-month cycle. Designed for the perimenopausal woman, providing effective relief of menopausal symptoms, reduced risk of osteoporosis and yet giving rise to periods only every 13 weeks. Periods are unlikely to be any heavier than normal, and 86% of women were still taking Tridestra at the end of the first year. The presentation and packaging of Tridestra is user-friendly, with 91 tablets in three blister packs, 70 tablets containing oestradiol valerate USP 2 mg, 14 tablets containing oestradiol valerate and medroxyprogesterone acetate and 7 placebo tablets.

## Fematrix

Fematrix (Solvay) is a transdermal patch delivering approximately 80 μg per 24 hours, 17 beta-oestradiol; one patch is applied twice weekly.

Indicated for the relief of menopausal symptoms in women with symptoms of oestrogen deficiency who have had a natural menopause or oöphorectomy. In women who still have a uterus, progestogen should be given for 12–14 days of each cycle.

'Smooth releasing, menopause easing, sweat cooling, flush soothing, slick fitting, secure sticking, quick peeling, great feeling, skin care, cost aware, new "spec", neat "n" discreet' (so the advert goes).

## Zumenon

Zumenon (Solvay) is a HRT containing oestradiol 2 mg and is taken once daily in tablet form for the relief of menopausal symptoms. Where necessary a progestogen should be given for 14 days of the cycle.

## Estring

Estring (Pharmaceia-Leiras) contains oestradiol in a silicone vaginal ring, administered only once every three months, offering a comfortable and convenient delivery of oestradiol into surrounding fluid and tissues to relieve local vaginal symptoms. As very little oestradiol reaches the systemic circulation, there is little chance of side-effects such as nausea and endometrial stimulation seen with systemic HRT. In trials patients have reported a higher level of acceptance of Estring than for vaginal cream.

## Oestrogel

Oestrogel (Hoechst Roussel) is a topical oestrogen replacement in a pressurized canister (see above).

## Kliofem

Kliofem (Novo Nordisk) is a period-free HRT for non-hysterectomized women, it should not be started earlier than one year after the last menstrual period when the risk of bleeding is unacceptably high. Kliofem is the first continuous combined HRT in the UK and is licensed for the treatment of menopausal symptoms and prophylaxis of osteoporosis. Continuous progestogen theoretically causes no withdrawal bleeds which may be more acceptable to women but irregular light bleeding is common, at least in the first six months of treatment.

## Lomexin

Lomexin (Upjohn) is a fenticonazole pessary for vaginal thrush. Fenticonazole pessaries are licenced for vulvovaginal candidiasis. They are as effective as clotrimazole at the higher strength. They are soft pliable pessaries which have been designed to be more comfortable than existing topical therapies. Some patients may require an applicator.

Fenticonazole is slightly more expensive than clotrimazole but less expensive than oral therapy.

## Contraception

### Mirena

Mirena (Pharmacia-Leiras) is a new development from the conventional IUCD, combining the benefits of both hormonal release and an IUCD. It acts differently to conventional IUCDs releasing levonorgestrel into the uterus at a rate of about 20 µg per day. Once inserted it is effective for up to three years.

It is said to be as effective contraceptively as sterilization, but is, of course, reversible. It does not result in heavy periods and there is a low risk of ectopic pregnancy and pelvic inflammatory disease (PID).

It is therefore suitable for some women who would be otherwise unsuitable candidates for an IUCD, namely, women with heavy periods or those at risk of PID or ectopic pregnancy.

It can also be used in perimenopausal women taking HRT, as the progestogen required to protect the uterus from hyperplasia.

Its effects are reversed within one month of removal. Unfortunately at present it costs nearly £100.

### Unipath personal contraceptive system

The user-effectiveness studies for this system are nearing completion; 1200 women were recruited to test it, and it is due to be launched in 1996.

The system offers objective analysis of the fertile phase using urine dip sticks which track the rise in oestrogen and the luteinizing hormone surge. An interval is added on to allow for ovulation and ovum life span. It is a hand held electronic monitor; the user presses a button each morning starting on day one of the period. A yellow light is a request for a urine dip stick test (16 will be required in the first cycle; eight in subsequent cycles). A red light indicates the fertile phase; a green light indicates days that are safe for unprotected intercourse. It is envisaged that the fertile days may be as few as eight, a significant reduction when compared with present natural family planning methods. The fertile phase can be defined as the combined duration of sperm survivability (3–5 days) plus ovum life span (24 hours).

Efficiency data is not yet available and the cost will be around £100 per person.

# 12: Contraception

Contraceptive advice is rarely a primary reason for referral to a gynaecologist, although the topic often arises during the course of gynaecological presentation. Training in family planning is an integral part of vocational training for general practitioners and the recently formed Faculty of Family Planning and Reproductive Health Care, part of the Royal College of Obstetricians and Gynaecologists, is a body set up to improve the standard of knowledge and training in reproductive medicine.

Whilst most newly qualified doctors have a basic knowledge of good contraceptive practice, there are many situations which arise in primary care where accurate detailed knowledge is essential, which drugs interfere with the pill for example and are they different for the combined pill and the progesterone-only pill (POP)?

Changes and new developments are occurring in all areas of family planning, from newer hormonal preparations to recently developed contraceptive implants, to progestogen-releasing intrauterine contraceptive devices (IUCDs). There has also been an increased interest in depot contraception which has lead to the licensing of Depo-Provera as a first line contraceptive in appropriate circumstances.

New products are also considered in Chapter 11 on New Developments in Gynaecology. See page 99.

For failure rates of all types of contraception see Table 12.1.

## Hormonal methods

### Combined oral contraceptive pill (COC)

The COC pill has been available for more than 20 years. It is used in the UK by more than 3 million women and has a low

**Table 12.1** Contraceptive failure rates.

| Method | Failure rate per 100 woman years |
|---|---|
| Sterilization (male and female) | 0.01–0.5 |
| Depo-Provera | 0.01–0.5 |
| Mirena | 0.2–0.5 |
| Norplant | 0.01–1 |
| Combined oral contraceptive pill | 0.2–3 |
| Progesterone-only pill (safer over age 35 years) | 0.34–4 |
| IUCD | 1–3 |
| Cap | 5–20 |
| Condom (male and female) | 5–15 |
| Natural methods | 6–25 |
| PC4 | 2–4 |
| Post-coital IUCD | <1 |

failure rate of less than 1 per 100 woman years. The pill combines ethinyloestradiol with a progestogen, the oldest of which are norethisterone and levonorgestrel, the newest desogestrel, gestodene and norgestimate. Its mechanism of action is the suppression of ovulation.

The COC pill is ideally suited to women up to the age of 35 years, or up to the age of 40 years in non-smokers.

One combined pill uses the oestrogen mestranol, whilst all the remaining combined pills contain ethinyl oestradiol, combined with norethisterone.

At the time of this publication, adverse publicity has surrounded the safety of COCs containing the progestogens, gestodene and desogestrel, because of the reported twofold increase risk of venous thrombo-embolism. The same studies did not show any increased risk of myocardial infarction or stroke. As a result, the Committee on the Safety of Medicines advised that COCs containing gestodene or desogestrel should not be used by women with risk factors for venous thrombo-embolism including obesity (defined as a body mass index (BMI) of $>30\,\text{kg/m}^2$), varicose veins or a previous history of thrombosis from any cause. Combined oral contraceptives containing gestodene or desogestrel could still however be used by women without such risk factors who are intolerant of other COCs or are prepared to accept the increased risk of thrombo-embolism.

The older COCs containing norethisterone and levo-norgestrel are more progestogen-dominant and can therefore give rise to side-effects such as acne, vaginal dryness, amenorrhoea and loss of libido, whilst the newer preparations containing desogestrel, norgestimate or gestodene are more oes-trogen-dominant and can therefore give rise to side-effects such as headaches, breast tenderness, fluid retention and increased vaginal discharge. If these side-effects are present or a problem then a more progestogen-dominant pill may be appropriate whereas progestogen type side-effects may be helped by an oestrogen-dominant pill.

## Contraindications

*Cardiovascular*
- Arterial or venous thrombosis or embolism
- Angina and ischaemic heart disease
- Valvular heart disease
- Pulmonary hypertension
- Sickle-cell anaemia

*Hepatic*
- Abnormal liver function
- Cholestatic jaundice
- Liver adenoma
- Porphyria
- Infectious hepatitis

*Other conditions*
- Undiagnosed vaginal bleeding
- Pregnancy
- Trophoblastic disease

- Hormone dependent cancer

Special precautions may be required with hypertension, Raynaud's disease, diabetes, asthma, renal disease, multiple sclerosis. Certain drugs which may inter-react including phenytoin, carbamazepine, primidone, barbiturates, rifampicin, and broad-spectrum antibiotics.

### Enzyme-inducing drugs and the COC

Enzyme-inducing drugs, including particularly carbamazepine, barbiturates, phenytoin, primidone, rifampicin and griseofulvin (not sodium valproate (Epilim), lamotrigine or vigabatrin), require 50 μg of oestrogen such as Ovran 50, usually taken three double packs in a row followed by a shortened four-day pill-free interval. If break-through bleeding occurs on this regimen 80 μg should be given in the same 'tricycling' regimen.

Drugs which alter the metabolism and therefore reduce the contraceptive effectiveness of the COC and POP.
- Barbituates
- Phenytoin
- Primidone
- Rifampicin
- Griseofulvin
- Spironolactone

Drugs which do not alter the metabolism and therefore do not reduce contraceptive effectiveness of COC and POP.
- Sodium valporate
- Clonazepam
- Lamotrigine
- Vigabatrin

### Risk reduction with the COC

The COC however reduces the risk of the following conditions.
- Ovarian cysts and cancer of the ovary

- Endometriosis
- Benign breast disease
- Fibroids
- Ectopic pregnancy

### The COC and elective surgery

The following recommendations have been suggested for women awaiting surgery whilst taking the combined oral contraceptive pill.

| | |
|---|---|
| Minor surgery (excluding varicose veins) | Continue pill as normal |
| Intermediate surgery, e.g. breast lump, hernia | Individual patient choice |
| Major surgery including orthopaedic procedures and varicose vein surgery | Must stop pill six to eight weeks before surgery |

Patients undergoing emergency procedures will probably be administered heparin.

### Progestogen-only pill (POP) preparations

There are currently six POPs, either based on norethisterone or levonorgestrel.

The POP is ideal for women in whom the use of synthetic oestrogens is contraindicated, as well as older women and women who are breast-feeding. It is less effective contraceptively than the COC but nevertheless a good choice of contraception particularly in properly selected patients. It must be taken regularly, each day without a break, preferably at the same time of the day. It is most effective approximately three hours after swallowing it.

The main side-effects are irregular bleeding which may be prolonged although not usually heavy. In addition, if conception does occur whilst taking the minipill there is a relatively increased risk of an ectopic pregnancy.

The contraceptive efficacy of POPs may be reduced by enzyme-inducing drugs particularly carbamazepine, barbiturates, phenytoin, primidone, (not sodium valproate, vigabatrin or lamotrigine) rifampicin, griseofulvin and spironlactone. Therefore in patients taking the POP, for whom other methods are unsuitable or for those who are prepared to take the risk (the POP is not the ideal choice for someone taking enzyme-inducing drugs), the dose of the POP should be doubled, i.e. two tablets daily (not one), continuously, without a break.

*Antibiotics do not reduce the effectiveness of POPs as contraceptives.*

### Contraindications

Contraindications to the POP are not the same as for the COC, in particular the POP is ideally suited for: women over the age of 35 years who smoke; anyone with a specific contraindication to the COC such as thrombo-embolism; patients with diabetes, hypertension or obesity; patients with migraine or those lactating and finally patients with some specific chronic conditions which may be exacerbated by oestrogen, such as systemic lupus erythematosus (SLE), Crohn's disease and sickle cell disease.

The POP is, however, contraindicated in patients with a history of arterial disease or at high risk of arterial disease including hyperlipidaemia, pregnancy, undiagnosed vaginal bleeding and recent trophoblastic disease.

Relative contraindications to the POP include risk factors for arterial disease, breast cancer, liver disorders and a past history of functional ovarian cysts.

### The 'seven day rule' following missed pills

If a pill is forgotten, either a COC or a POP, or vomiting occurs whilst taking the pill or an enzyme-inducing drug is taken whilst taking the pill, particularly rifampicin, carbamazepine, barbiturates, phenytoin, primidone, (not sodium valproate, vigabatrin or lamotrigine) and griseofulvin, the 'seven day rule' of using an additional method of contraception for seven days after the event or illness which may render the pill ineffective, should be applied and explained to all pill-users.

If a COC is missed or is taken late by less than 12 hours, then there is no need to apply the above 'seven day rule' but if it is missed or late by more than 12 hours or any of the other circumstances apply then the 'seven day rule' is imperative. If the missed or forgotten pill occurs during the last seven days of the COC packet, then the next packet of COCs should be taken at the end of the current packet *without a break*, i.e. no seven pill-free days.

*Missed COCs at the beginning of a packet, i.e. after seven pill-free days, or at the end of a packet, thereby potentially extending the pill-free period to longer than seven days are most at risk of ovulation occurring.*

### The pill and amenorrhoea

*COC-users with absent withdrawal bleeds.* Provided that the patient is not pregnant, the oestrogen and progestogen are suppressing follicle-stimulating hormone (FSH) and luteinizing hormone (LH) in a normal way, but the uterus is not responding in a normal way by a 'withdrawal bleed'. The pill is working very satisfactorily and the woman is no more prone to post-pill amenorrhoea than any other patient. If the patient is not happy with this explanation and wants a monthly bleed to reassure her that all is well, then a pill higher in oestrogen or progestogen may be chosen.

*Absent periods, whilst taking the minipill.* Provided that pregnancy is excluded, this means that the pituitary/hypothalamus is particularly sensitive and that the POP is working very effectively. This patient should probably not take the COC in the future.

*Women requesting the pill who have a past history of unstable menstrual periods.* If they have had true amenorrhoea, for more than six months; or if they are underweight, they probably ought not to use hormonal contraception.

## Postcoital contraception

Emergency contraception, whether hormonal or by inserting an IUCD should never be used as a regular method of family planning but may be used in situations where other methods have not been used or have failed, e.g. a condom bursting or coming off the flaccid penis before it is properly withdrawn from the vagina.

Both methods of emergency contraception have been used in the UK for more than 10 years.

### The 'morning-after pill'

This term is misleading as it implies that hormonal postcoital contraception must be used the 'morning after' unprotected intercourse whereas the 'morning-after pill' is effective when given within 72 hours of unprotected intercourse.

*Schering PC4* is a specially packaged set of four pills each containing 50 µg ethinyloestradiol. The first two pills must be taken within 72 hours of unprotected intercourse followed by the remaining two pills exactly 12 hours later. In the event of Schering PC4 not being available, two 50 µg pills such as Ovran 50 may be substituted.

The postcoital pill works by preventing ovulation (if taken early enough in the cycle) or rendering the endometrium unfavourable for implantation and impeding the passage of eggs along the fallopian tubes.

Nausea is commonly reported as a side-effect although vomiting rarely occurs. If it is thought likely that vomiting may occur an anti-emetic may be given with PC4 or alternatively, two extra 50 µg pills can be given with instructions to take them if vomiting occurs within two hours of taking either of the two PC4 tablets.

After taking PC4 the next menstrual period usually occurs at or around the normal expected time of the next period. The patient should be asked to report to the doctor if the next period is delayed by more than a few days or does not appear at all.

If a patient requiring PC4 is taking enzyme-inducing drugs, particularly carbamazepine, barbiturates, phenytoin, primidone, spironolactone and griseofulvin, or for patients taking a broad-spectrum antibiotic, three PC4 tablets should be given followed by three tablets 12 hours later. Treating patients on combined pills who are taking antibiotics and make an error in the 'extra precautions' regimen, still give three PC4 tablets and repeat the dose 12 hours later and offer this same regimen both whilst the patient is actually taking the antibiotic and for the seven days after taking the antibiotic, *even if the antibiotic is taken in the pill-free week.* Antibiotics affect the pill in approximately one in 250 women, but even though the risk is relatively small, if a pregnancy results following wrong advice, medico-legally the practitioner would be indefensible.

*Rifampicin* is an extremely potent enzyme-inducer (it is most commonly used not only in the treatment of TB but also in prophylaxis against meningococcal meningitis) and if PC4 is used the dose should be *doubled*, i.e. four PC4 tablets followed by four more tablets 12 hours later.

If a woman who is breast-feeding requests the morning-after pill, there is no contraindication and no need to discard milk, after administration of PC4 though she may prefer to do so for 24 hours. A woman who is fully breast-feeding, fully amenorrhoeic and not yet six months postpartum is at very low risk of conception even without using any specific method.

Where the combined pill is totally contraindicated, 6 mg levonorgestrel (20 Microval or Norgeston tablets) may be given in one stat dose, within 12 hours of unprotected intercourse. If neither method is acceptable, and the risk of pregnancy is significant, insertion of an IUCD should be considered.

## The emergency IUCD

A copper containing IUCD may be inserted in the usual way and is effective as a postcoital method of contraception provided it is fitted within five days of unprotected intercourse, or up to five days after the earliest calculated ovulation day in the cycle in question, e.g. up to day 19 in a regular 28-day cycle. The newer progestogen-releasing Mirena is *not* recommended as postcoital contraception.

The IUCD produces endometrial changes whilst the copper inhibits enzymes involved in fertilization and implantation.

Only four documented failures have been reported. It is the most effective method of postcoital contraception.

Side-effects are the same as for IUCDs in general. The insertion of an IUCD can be a painful procedure particularly for someone who has never been pregnant. It is common therefore for women to have a little bleeding and some discomfort for a few days after insertion.

If a woman is at high risk of pelvic infection, screening for sexually transmitted diseases (STDs) particularly *Chlamydia* should be considered as should referral to the local genito-urinary medicine clinic. Antibiotic cover may be worthwhile considering where screening is unavailable or not practical.

*Contraindications.* An IUCD must not be inserted if a woman is pregnant, has undiagnosed genital bleeding or current pelvic infection. A coil should not be used if avoidable where there is a past history of ectopic pregnancy, and the Yuzpe method would be preferable. Intrauterine contraceptive devices should also be avoided in patients on immunosuppressive therapy including corticosteroids for fear of silent infection.

Care must be taken when advising the following groups in the use of an IUCD.

- Nulliparous patients (particularly under the age of 20 years).
- Those with particularly heavy or painful periods.
- Those with valvular heart disease (probably require antibiotic cover if a coil is inserted).
- Those with a past history of pelvic infection.
- Those with diabetes.
- Those with an abnormal (including fibroids) uterus.
- Endometriosis.
- Wilson's disease.
- Penicillamine treatment.

## Barrier methods

### *Male condom*

Condoms are made of natural latex rubber. Their correct usage gives rise to a low failure rate of less than two per 100 woman years. It is recommended that condoms are used with spermicides for greater protection. Their only drawback is occasional sensitivity to the rubber, but non-allergenic forms are available.

Apart from their contraceptive benefit they are also beneficial in reducing STDs.

### *Female condom*

Femidom is sold over the counter but is not freely available on prescription. They can be obtained free from family planning clinics. They are biologically inert, much bigger than the male condom and sometimes their appearance is a little off-putting, but for some women they are highly acceptable and effectively fill a gap in contraception. Femidom requires no medical supervision, no spermicide and no special fitting.

## Diaphragms, caps and sponges

Diaphragms and caps are available free on prescription. Vaginal sponges are not. They are all barrier methods which occlude the cervical canal. They are suitable for women comfortable with handling the genital area and are inserted before intercourse commences, unlike male condoms which interrupt intercourse. They should be used in conjunction with spermicides; the contraceptive sponge has a spermicide incorporated within it.

The disadvantage of diaphragms and caps is that they have to be correctly fitted by trained medical staff and checked after initial prescribing to ensure a good fit and technique of insertion. Caps are more suitable for women with poor muscular tone or uterovaginal prolapse.

The *vaginal sponge* comes in one size only so it does not require medical supervision. Unfortunately it has a high failure rate unlike the diaphragm and cap which have a failure rate similar to the male condom of about two per 100 woman years.

All of these devices must be left in inside the vagina for at least six hours after intercourse.

As barrier methods they may offer some protection against STDs and possibly carcinoma of the cervix.

## Intrauterine contraceptive devices (IUCDs)

Newer IUCDs have been developed which can be left in place for longer than the usual five years for Multiload 375 and Novagard and Nova-T. Ortho-Gyne T 380 S is now licenced for eight years.

Intrauterine contraceptive devices are not usually recommended for use by nulliparous patients and may not be ideal for those women with multiple sexual partners because of the increased risk of infection.

Side-effects of the IUCD are heavier prolonged periods, an

increased risk of pelvic infection and a relatively increased risk of ectopic pregnancy.

### Contraindications

An IUCD must not be inserted if a woman is pregnant, has undiagnosed genital bleeding or current pelvic infection. A coil should not be used if avoidable where there is a past history of ectopic pregnancy, and the Yuzpe method would be preferable. Intrauterine contraceptive devices should also be avoided in patients on immunosuppressive thereapy including corticosteroids for fear of silent infection.

Care must be taken when advising the following groups in the use of an IUCD.

- Nulliparous patients (particularly under the age of 20 years).
- Those with particularly heavy or painful periods.
- Those with valvular heart disease (probably require antibiotic cover if a coil is inserted).
- Those with a past history fo pelvic infection.
- Those with diabetes.
- Those with an abnormal (including fibroids) uterus.
- Endometriosis.
- Wilson's disease.
- Penicillamine treatment.

### Mirena

Mirena is a new development from the conventional IUCD, combining the benefits of both hormonal contraception and an IUCD. It acts differently to conventional IUCDs releasing levonorgestrel into the uterus at a rate of about 20 µg per day. Once inserted, usually within seven days of the onset of menstruation, or six weeks postpartum, it is effective for up to three years, although it is hoped that the licence will be extended to five years.

The levonorgestrel is contained in a reservoir in the vertical stem and is released at approximately 20μg per day (equivalent to two POPs per week).

It is said to be as effective contraceptively as sterilization, but is of course reversible, it does not result in heavy periods and there is a low risk of ectopic pregnancy and pelvic inflammatory disease (PID).

The device usually causes reduced menstrual blood flow and a significant proportion of users become oligo- or amenorrhoeic, which can cause concern regarding pregnancy. Twenty per cent of women become amenorrhoeic after one year's use.

It is therefore suitable for some women who would be otherwise unsuitable candidates for an IUCD, namely, women with heavy periods or those at risk of PID or ectopic pregnancy.

It can also be used in perimenopausal women taking hormone replacement therapy (HRT), as the progestogen is required to protect the uterus from hyperplasia. Its effects are reversed within one month of removal, making the possibility of an early pregnancy much more likely than with other long-acting contraceptives.

Unfortunately at present it costs nearly £100, therefore it is probably best reserved for women who have heavy periods or in whom the ordinary coil may otherwise be contraindicated (see above). There is insufficient information on its use in nulliparous women and, as with other IUCDs, its use in this group cannot be recommended.

## Depot injections

*Depo-Provera* (depot medroxyprogesterone acetate 150mg) and *Noristerat* (norethisterone oenanthate 200mg) are both highly effective contraceptives given by intramuscular injection once every 12 weeks (for Depo-Provera) or every 8 weeks (for Noristerat). They are particularly suitable for women where oestrogen is contraindicated or for women who are unreliable taking pills or find other methods unsuitable. They may also be useful for women with premenstrual syndrome, fibrocystic breast disease or endometriosis.

Common side-effects are amenorrhoea, which is common particularly in women using the method for a year or more, weight gain and occasionally backache. Fertility may be delayed on stopping the method.

### Administration of Depo-Provera

Depot injections are usually given on the first day of the cycle and as such are safe, contraceptively, immediately. The depot injection can be given up to the fifth day of the cycle but if not given on the first day, alternative precautions should be used for the first seven days.

The injection site should not be rubbed after administration as this may adversely affect release of the hormone.

If the woman is postpartum and not breast-feeding, the first injection should be given within five days of delivery. In breast-feeding women, the injection should, if possible, be delayed until five weeks after delivery. Early administration in both breast-feeding and non-breast-feeding women is associated with increased menstrual irregularity. If the first injection is given later than three weeks after delivery, in a non-breast-feeding woman, extra precautions should be used for the first seven days. Depo-Provera can normally be given within five days of a miscarriage or abortion without the need for extra precautions.

*Subsequent injections* should be given 12 weeks later and no later than 13 weeks after the previous injection. If the next dose is late by three days beyond 13 weeks since the last injection then PC4 plus an immediate injection of Depo-Provera is acceptable. If the next dose is late by five days beyond 13 weeks since the last injection, it would be acceptable contraceptively to fit an IUCD and give the next Depo-Provera immediately, but counselling must take place on the very low risk of potential harm to a fetus and follow-up must take place three weeks later to exclude pregnancy.

### Changing from the COC to Depo-Provera

If the patient is in the first five tablet-free days, an injection of Depo-Provera will give her immediate cover.

If the patient is at day six onwards in her cycle, following an injection of Depo-Provera, she should be advised to take additional precautions such as using a barrier method of contraception, for the next 14 days.

If a further depot injection is requested after a longer gap than 13 weeks plus three or five days (see above) then abstinence or the use of a barrier method of contraception for 14 days should be advised, a pregnancy test carried out and if negative, then the next injection may be given.

In patients who are taking enzyme-inducing drugs, particularly carbamazepine, barbiturates, phenytoin, primidone, rifampicin and griseofulvin (but not sodium valproate (Epilim)) the interval between injections should be reduced to 10 weeks.

### Bleeding problems whilst taking Depo-Provera

Whilst receiving Depo-Provera, although amenorrhoea usually occurs after several injections, menstrual disturbances, including too frequent bleeding, can occur and may be treated in one of two ways. The next injection may be given early, as soon as eight weeks since the previous injection. Alternatively, a short course of oestrogen, such as Premarin, or a short course of the COC (if not contraindicated) may be given.

### Contraindications

Contraindications for an injectable progestogen are similar to those for the POP; i.e. in patients with a history of arterial disease or at high risk of arterial disease including hyperlipidaemias, pregnancy, undiagnosed vaginal bleeding and recent trophoblastic disease.

Relative contraindications to the POP include risk factors for arterial disease, breast cancer, liver disorders and a past history of functional ovarian cysts.

Unlike the POP, Depo-Provera is highly suitable for women who have a history of ectopic pregnancy or ovarian cysts.

*Depo-Provera and bone density.* Conflicting evidence suggests that there may be a reduction in bone density following long-term Depo-Provera usage, but this is quite reversible, provided that the woman stops using Depo-Provera prior to the menopause.

Those women most at risk of osteoporosis, e.g. positive family history, smokers, low body mass index, sedentary lifestyle and those who have had prolonged periods of amenorrhoea, should be counselled accordingly.

Women reaching the menopause whilst on Depo-Provera should be considered for HRT to prevent loss of bone mass; for women who have been taking Depo-Provera long-term and who have a low serum oestradiol of less than 150pmol/l, it may be worth considering alternative methods of contraception. Normal levels of serum oestradiol are a relatively reassuring indication that Depo-Provera may be continued.

## Prolonged bleeding following cessation of Depo-Provera

One of the commonest side-effects incurred upon stopping the use of Depo-Provera for contraception is prolonged menstrual blood loss. Usually, with reassurance, this will settle with no specific treatment required. Sometimes, however, the patient is keen to try to conceive and requests 'something to clear it up'. In these circumstances, first check the serum beta-human chorionic gonadotrophin (HCG) to exclude an ectopic pregnancy. Then prescribe medroxyprogesterone acetate (Depo-Provera) 10mg to be taken three times a day for one week. A 'period' will then follow, but a normal cycle pattern should establish itself afterwards. If this is not the case referral to a gynaecologist for endometrial sampling or dilatation and curettage (D&C) is necessary.

## Norplant

More than 14000 women in the UK, and 3 million women worldwide use this method of long-term progestogen-only contraception, which is delivered from six matchstick-sized silastic capsules inserted intradermally, usually into the upper arm, providing contraception for five years. There will soon be a newer version comprising of only two rods.

Norplant is a highly effective contraceptive being nearly 100% effective in the first two years and 98% effective over the five years.

Norplant is intended for long-term contraception, particularly in women aged between 18–40 years, it is effective for five years. It is important in counselling to highlight potential side-effects before proceeding with insertion (see below). The most common side-effect is menstrual disturbance, scanty blood loss is not uncommon and does not require treatment but heavy or prolonged blood loss may be best managed by taking one packet of the combined oral contraceptive pill to provoke endometrial proliferation.

*Local reactions* following implantation include irritation at the site of insertion occurring at variable times following insertion, and is one of the commonest side-effects. Correct aseptic procedure reduces the risk. One per cent of women have Norplant removed because of arm pain. Other common side-effects are irregular bleeding and headache.

Other unwanted side-effects may occur such as weight gain, breast tenderness, acne, nausea, dizziness, increased or decreased hair growth. Disruption of ovulation may cause an increase in benign ovarian cysts.

The contraceptive efficacy of implants may be reduced by enzyme-inducing drugs particularly carbamazepine, barbiturates, phenytoin, primidone, rifampicin, griseofulvin and spironolactone. Antibiotics do not reduce the effectiveness of progestogens as contraceptives.

Because of the mode of action (see below) there is a possible increased risk of ectopic pregnancy, as there is with other progestogen-only forms of contraception, although this is less than POPs because of the higher overall effectiveness of Norplant.

The ideal time for insertion of Norplant is on day one of the menstrual cycle in which case contraception is immediate. If Norplant is inserted up to the fifth day of the cycle additional contraception such as condoms should be used for the next seven days. At other times in the cycle Norplant may still be inserted provided pregnancy has reliably been excluded and condoms are used for the next seven days. Postnatal insertion may be carried out 21 days after delivery and no extra precautions are required. Norplant is inserted under local anaesthetic.

Patients are usually followed-up three months after insertion and annually thereafter, mainly to enquire into bleeding pattern.

Norplant should be removed after five years, again under local anaesthetic. Removal can be a more difficult procedure than insertion.

Within general practice there is no separate fee for insertion of Norplant although the FP1001 should be completed in the usual manner.

Norplant causes suppression of ovulation in about 50% of cycles and interferes with the surge of LH as well as inhibiting implantation.

### Side-effects of Norplant and their management (Table 12.2)

*Contraindications* to depot progesterone (Norplant and Depo-Provera) are the same as for the POP and are not the same as for the oestrogen containing combination oral contraceptive (COC), in particular the *depot progesterone* is ideally suited for women over the age of 35 years who smoke, anyone with a specific contraindication to the COC such as thromboembolism, patients with diabetes, hypertension or obesity, patients with migraine, those lactating and finally patients with some specific chronic conditions which may be exacerbated by oestrogen, such as SLE, Crohn's disease and sickle cell disease.

**Table 12.2** Side-effects of Norplant and their management.

| Side-effect | Management |
| --- | --- |
| Heavy or prolonged periods | One cycle of the COC |
| Acne | Treat as usual, e.g. antibiotic |
| Weight gain | Dietary advice |
| Mood swings | No specific treatment |
| Headache | Treat symptomatically |

*Depot progesterone is, however, contraindicated* in patients with a history of arterial disease or at high risk of arterial disease including hyperlipidaemia, pregnancy, undiagnosed vaginal bleeding and recent trophoblastic disease.

Relative contraindications to the progesterone include risk factors for arterial disease, breast cancer, liver disorders and a past history of functional ovarian cysts.

## Vaginal rings

Vaginal rings as a form of contraception are not widely used or available in this country though popular in some others. There are two types, one containing both oestrogen and progesterone, which is inserted and left *in situ* for three weeks, and one containing progesterone only, which is inserted and left *in situ* for three months.

They work in the same way as tablets but have the advantage that they are not affected by gastro-intestinal absorption.

### Contraception and confidentiality for patients under the age of 16 years

Young patients under the age of 16 are said to fear seeking contraception, particularly from their family GP because they are uncertain of their rights to confidentiality.

It is estimated that of the estimated 52000 sexually active 15-year-old females in England in 1991, only 18000 visited family planning clinics, some visited their own GPs, whilst many others visited neither.

*Young people, regardless of their age, are entitled to their rights of confidentiality.*

If the young person is asking for contraception, the following issues must be addressed and recorded in their medical notes.

1 They are competent to be able to understand and give their consent.

2 They have been recommended to discuss their choice with their parents.

3 They are likely to have a sexual relationship whether their request for contraception is accepted or refused.

4 They need contraceptive advice to prevent their physical or mental health suffering as a result.

5 It is in their best interests to have contraception even without parental consent if necessary.

Following these guidelines is imperative for medico-legal reasons, but as long as the guidelines are followed the practitioner is within his or her rights to give contraception in the same way as for a person over the age of 16 years.

It is always worth discussing safe sex and demonstrating the use of condoms and promoting their usage even if the pill is chosen as the method of contraception.

The author usually points out to the young girl that it is technically illegal for a man to have sex with a girl under the age of 16 years, but of course confidentiality will be respected.

Finally, it is also worthwhile enquiring tactfully who the

partner is. Occasionally it can be a much older male, including a close relative, and the girl may need a greater deal of support particularly from outside agencies such as social services.

## Contraception and the menopause

Some form of contraception is usually recommended as necessary for at least one year after the final menstrual period if this occurs after the age of 50 or for two years after the last menstrual period if this occurs under the age of 50. Problems can arise however in giving advice on the continuing need for contraception after the menopause if the woman is taking the COC or the POP or HRT at the time of the menopause as these may continue to give rise to 'periods' or withdrawal bleeds well after the time that ovulation has ceased.

In women taking the COC at the time of the menopause, whilst ovarian failure and eventual cessation still occurs, symptoms of oestrogen deficiency will be masked by the pill. Diagnosis of the menopause can be achieved by stopping the COC and, if amenorrhoea follows, together with symptoms of the menopause and a raised FSH on two separate occasions, this is strongly suggestive of the menopause.

In women who are taking the POP and still having periods at the time of the menopause, there is no need to stop the pill as progesterone does not influence FSH, therefore a raised FSH, whilst still taking the minipill is diagnostic of the menopause. If a woman who is taking the POP is amenorrhoeic but has a normal FSH then the amenorrhoea is pill-induced, *and is not indicative that the menopause has occurred*.

In women under the age of 50 years, it is best to measure the FSH on two separate occasions separated by three months if contraception is to be stopped completely on reaching the menopause and simple non-hormonal contraception used for 12 months for absolute safety.

*Women reaching the menopause and taking HRT* will still

get a rise in FSH, despite the small dose of exogenous oestrogen but this is a less reliable indicator of being able to stop using some form of contraception.

Barrier methods may be less acceptable as an alternative method of contraception, around the time of the menopause, due either to vaginal dryness or erectile dysfunction.

The IUCD may be a very acceptable form of contraception for the older woman and any device fitted after the age of 40 years can probably be left *in situ* until one year after the menopause or until the age of 53 years if the woman is taking HRT.

Sterilization, by one or other partner has often been chosen as a method before the menopause has been reached.

Low-dose COC or POP are acceptable and safe up to the menopause provided that no contraindications to either exist.

## Sterilization

Sterilization, both male and female, is the final and safest step towards preventing pregnancy that a couple can make. Often the GP is in the most critical and knowledgeable position in helping a couple to decide that this method is suitable for them. After referral by the GP the couple will usually be counselled by the specialist who is likely to perform the operation, but careful selection of patients and provision of information by the GP may prevent an inappropriate referral or even an inappropriate request. It is always wisest to avoid referral for sterilization at a time of some crisis for the couple. Sterilization rarely 'solves problems' in fact it can often make family matters worse if done inappropriately.

It is essential with both forms of sterilization to emphasize that the procedures are designed to be irreversible. In exceptional circumstances, for example following the death of a former spouse and remarriage to a new partner who wants children, reversal may be attempted.

Both forms of sterilization have a small but real failure rate. In counselling for sterilization, male or female, complications, such as wound infections and failure rates should be discussed (see below). Also, consideration of suitability for local procedures should be determined, e.g. if the local surgeon or GP normally performs vasectomies under a local anaesthetic, then a man who may be more suitable for the procedure under general anaesthetic, e.g. an absent testicle, should not be referred for a vasectomy under a local anaesthetic.

Psychosexual problems in either partner should be addressed prior to sterilization.

### Female sterilization

Female sterilization is usually performed laparoscopically under a general anaesthetic, allowing the patient to go home the same or the following day, provided there are no complications.

The effect of the operation is immediate and the woman is usually back to normal activities within 48 hours.

Immediate postoperative complications are rare but postoperative pain can be severe, nausea and vomiting may occur and intra-abdominal accidents, such as bowel perforation can rarely occur. In the longer term, women who have had a laparoscopic sterilization may suffer from heavier periods, possibly resulting in an increased rate of hysterectomy, although this is controversial and may simply be the effect of the woman stopping taking the oral contraceptive pill which she may have employed for some years.

Laparoscopic female sterilization is most often performed using Filshie clips, which have a failure rate of 1 in 1000 applications, although diathermy may be employed. In the event of pregnancy occurring following sterilization, ectopic pregnancy is slightly more likely to occur.

Ideally, all sterilizations should be performed in the first 10 days of the menstrual cycle to prevent a possible pregnancy occurring in the luteal phase. If this rule cannot be applied then alternative contraception should be employed prior to the operation. If an IUCD has been used as contraception prior to sterilization then it is probably safest and wisest to leave it *in situ* until after the first period following the sterilization procedure.

## *Male sterilization*

Vasectomy is usually performed under a local anaesthetic through bilateral incisions overlying the vas deferens, the procedure lasting 10–15 minutes. Some swelling, bruising and attendant discomfort is to be expected and may last for several days. The patient can usually go home immediately following the procedure, although it is probably wise that he does not drive himself home. For the first few days wearing a scrotal support or a tight-fitting pair of underpants may be helpful and avoidance of strenuous physical activity is advised particularly, for example, cycling or horseback riding.

The decision to return to work after the operation will depend on the individual and on the individual's work but the author usually advises two days off work under any circumstances.

Immediate complications are rare but include haematoma, which occasionally will require drainage, and infection.

A discharging wound occurring up to 10 days following the operation is quite common and is best managed with salt water baths. Antibiotics are rarely indicated.

Two separated sperm counts are usually required from a masturbation sample following the operation, usually around three months after the operation. If sperm are found to be present further samples will be required until two consecutive samples are negative. Positive tests six months following the operation should result in the patient being referred back for possible further surgery. *Even after two consecutive negative sperm counts there is still a very small risk of failure* of the procedure to prevent pregnancy and this should be emphasized.

Chronic pain following vasectomy is unusual but does occur and may be helped by taking non-steroidal anti-inflammatory drugs (NSAIDs) until the situation usually subsides spontaneously. If, however, pain persists further surgery to remove nerve fibres trapped during the operation may be necessary.

Suggestions have been made of an association between vasectomy and renal stones, cancers of the testis and prostate, though there is no conclusive evidence of any of these.

Finally, in counselling for vasectomy, it is important to enquire into any allergy to local anaesthetic, bleeding tendencies or local genital disorders.

## Sperm banking

Occasionally patients wish to 'hedge their bets' by freeze-storing their sperm in a sperm bank for some years following their operation. The British Pregnancy Advisory Service provides this service privately for a relatively small fee. One in 10 men with a relatively low sperm count are unsuitable as their sperm cannot survive the process of freezing and thawing.

## Questions

**Q1**: Which COC pills have been implicated in recent research claiming that they increase the risk of thrombo-embolism, and are they totally contraindicated in everyone?

**A**: COC preparations containing the newer progestogens, gestodene and desogestrel, namely, Femodene, Femodene ED, Marvelon, Mercilon, Minulet, Tri-Minulet and Triadene have been reported to show a twofold increase in the risk of thrombo-embolism compared with combined pills containing the older progestogens, norethisterone and levonorgestrel.

The Committee on Safety of Medicines has therefore recommended that the above pills are not given to any woman with risk factors for thrombo-embolism, namely, obesity (defined as a BMI $>30\,kg/m^2$, varicose veins or a previous history of thrombosis from any cause). Combined oral contraceptive pills containing gestodene or desogestrel may however be prescribed for women with no contraindications who are intolerant of other COC preparations or prepared to accept the increased risk of thrombo-embolism.

The safety of the other 'new' progestogen, norgestimate (Cilest), has not been implicated in the recent research findings.

Myocardial infarction and stroke are other rare but important risks of COCs, but no evidence has been found to suggest that the risk of these is increased with combined pills containing gestodene or desogestrel.

**Q2**: When will a male contraceptive be available?

**A**: Trials of testosterone injections which reduce gonadotrophins whilst maintaining virility and libido, are underway although there is concern about the theoretical increased risk of coronary heart disease and prostatic cancer.

**Q3**: If conception does occur with an IUCD *in situ*, should it be removed and when?

**A**: There is a reduction in the risk of miscarriage from 50% to 25% with the early removal of the IUCD. As the gravid uterus enlarges the threads become drawn up making it impossible and dangerous to try to attempt to remove the device. It should therefore be removed as soon as possible, if the threads are visible, although if difficulty is encountered it should be left *in situ*.

**Q4**: Should the combined pill be stopped at the age of 35 years in woman who smoke?

**A**: Probably yes. Cigarettes are one of the most important risk factors for heart and arterial disease, and when combined with taking the oral contraceptive pill, the risk of fatal myocardial infarct may be increased by up to 21 times. Pill-related deaths in smokers rise from 1 in 10000 for women aged 34 years or less, to 1 in 550 for women over the age of 45 years old. Therefore smokers over the age of 35 years should change to an alternative method of contraception.

# Bibliography

Guillebaud, J. (1985) The Contraceptive pill and your operation. *British Medical Journal* **291**, 498–499.

Guillebaud, J. (1994) *Contraception. Your Questions Answered*. Churchill Livingstone, Singapore.

Ironside, V. & Biggs S. (1995) *The Subfertility Handbook*. Sheldon Press.

Mason, M-C (1993) *Male infertility – Men Talking*. Routledge.

Neuberg R. (1994) *Infertility*. Thorsons.

# Index